# Hidden

# Health

# Secrets

# Acknowledgements

Several people gave their time and energy to help me write this book. Special thanks to:

...  Janice McCall Failes who researched and drafted part of the initial manuscript. Your patience and dedication is appreciated.

...  Cheryl Daly and Linda Sciullo for your typing and proofreading.

...  Kip Marshall for your artwork.

...  My wife, Gayle, for your encouragement and the editing of the manuscript.

...  All the supportive staff of FC&A, for their willingness to help in every way.

...  But most of all, our thanks and praise is for our Lord and Saviour, who loves us, supports us and guides us.

Do you not know that your body is the temple —
the very sanctuary — of the Holy Spirit Who lives
within you, Whom you have received (as a Gift)
from God? You are not your own, You were
bought for a price — purchased with a
preciousness and paid for, made His own. So
then, honor God and bring glory to Him in your
body.

— 1 Corinthians 6:19 - 20 Amplified

# Table Of Contents

# Introduction

Recently, scientists have discovered many natural ways to help restore your health. Some of these secrets have been known for many years as folk medicine, home remedies, or simply the advice given to others by people who are extraordinarily healthy.

Aches, pains, health problems and diseases are facts of life. True, we are all going to have health problems, but have you ever wondered why some people are almost never sick? Many of these healthy people know and practice health secrets that keep them feeling good. Some individuals practice them consciously; others, perhaps only by accident or because of environmental circumstances.

Staying healthy may be overcoming something that seems small like leg cramps or tiredness... or it may be preventing something threatening to your overall health... like cancer or diabetes. This new book, Hidden Health Secrets, reveals hundreds of natural healing secrets. It shows you how to relieve or prevent many health problems.

The book also mentions certain standard medical treatments like drugs and surgery. Medical treatment shouldn't be ignored, but natural prevention or treatment may help too.

Standard treatments are mentioned for comparison to determine if natural methods of prevention and treatment may in some cases be better. For example, high blood pressure can be treated by many natural methods or with drugs prescribed by doctors. In many cases, both methods can reduce high blood pressure, but natural methods which work are a good alternative if your doctor agrees, because they avoid the unpleasant side effects of prescription drugs.

## What Works and What Doesn't Work

The health secrets in this book are not guaranteed to succeed with everyone. For example, there are many things that people can do to minimize wrinkles. Nevertheless, wrinkling of the skin is something which will occur to a greater or lesser extent as people age, no matter what they do.

Dietary fiber can help to avoid the "laxative trap" and relieve constipation naturally as well as prevent many other diseases. Unfortunately, if a person takes a strong prescription drug like codeine, which has constipation as a side effect, even large amounts of bran may not be enough to prevent constipation, and a laxative may be necessary.

As I wrote this book, I realized that I could not pass judgment on the effectiveness of most health secrets that I discovered. Some of these secrets may work for you but not for other people. Some may work for other people but not for you. Many of the health secrets reported in this book may be controversial or unproven by controlled scientific studies. I've simply reported the ideas in this book, because there is some evidence that they have worked for some people. In doing this, I have attempted to separate fact from fiction and to give special attention to health secrets which have been confirmed by scientific research. I have attempted, wherever possible, to verify the accuracy of information reported in this book. Nevertheless, since these are reports of the research of other people, I cannot guarantee their safety or effectiveness.

Mark Twain once made a joke about people who uncritically accept every health tip they read in print. He said that he wondered how many people had had problems as a result of typographical errors.

Because of the possibility of errors in reporting the research of others and because medical science is such a rapidly expanding field with new developments reported each day, I ask that you consult carefully with your own physician before trying any of the health tips listed in this book.

It can be dangerous to rely on self-treatment or home remedies and neglect proven medical treatments, such as surgery in cases of cancer. A good physician is the best judge of what sort of medical treatment may be needed for certain diseases. It's good to choose a physician who is open-minded about safe, natural methods of prevention and treatment.

# Acne

Common acne is caused by hormone imbalances combined with a diet which is high in saturated fats and sugar or refined starches like white flour. Acne is uncommon among primitive people who eat a diet which is low in fat or sugar and moderate in calories. Acne begins when glands in the skin produce excessive amounts of oil. Next, this oily skin is supplied with high levels of sugar in the bloodstream and in perspiration under the influence of androgenic hormones ("male" hormones which are also found in lower levels in females), which are produced in excessive amounts, starting in many children during puberty. Finally, bacteria thrive in skin pores and cause the eruptions characteristic of acne.

As an illustration of how acne is related to modern diets, acne used to be unknown to Eskimos who traditionally have eaten a diet mainly of game and fish. About thirty years ago, Eskimos began to become more westernized in eating and living habits. Today, teenage Eskimos who have grown up on much the same diet as other American teenagers, have a high prevalence of acne. Many Eskimos blame their acne on soda pop, candy and high-fat processed foods that they eat. Studies of the traditional Eskimo diet indicate that it was extremely low in carbohydrates and moderately low in fat.

Acne usually breaks out first in the early teenage years among susceptible children who have large increases in androgenic hormones both among boys and girls. It can be prevented by eating a moderate calorie diet which is high in fiber and very low in saturated fat, sugar and refined carbohydrates like white flour as well as by substituting foods like cold water fish, which are very high in polyunsaturated oils for meat or poultry products.

However, once acne has taken hold in susceptible individuals, it may not be gotten rid of quickly with a change in diet. The best modern medical treatment involves application of benzoyl peroxide solution or cream to the skin. Many topical preparations containing benzoyl peroxide are sold over the counter in drug stores. Another medical treatment involves the administration of a prescription drug called Accutane®. Unfortunately, there are serious side effects associated with this drug, including a high incidence of birth defects among pregnant women who have taken it early in pregnancy. One study reported an incidence of birth defects as high as 30% among users of this drug who were pregnant.

Once acne has been controlled, diet can play a large role in keeping it from recurring. Since acne sufferers tend to be overweight, even the best dietary management may fail if people overload their systems with excessive calories which may circulate in the bloodstream as sugar and fat. Dietary management should include restrictions on overeating as well as a good selection of low-fat, low-sugar food.

### Alcoholism

Alcoholism occurs when people drink alcohol regularly to the extent that it affects their health. Some people can become alcoholics without ever being noticeably drunk, but other alcoholics frequently go on binges where they drink so much that they pass out.

Alcoholism is a disease of the spirit, the will, the mind and the body. The first step towards control of the illness is a determination on the part of the alcoholic that he wants to be cured and that he is willing to endure the physical hardships of withdrawal from alcohol. Once that decision is made, the best procedure is to get help by withdrawing from alcohol in a hospital where there are physical barriers preventing the alcoholic from having second thoughts and once again returning to alcohol.

After a few weeks, the recovering alcoholic, when he's released, will be greatly helped by joining a group like Alcoholics Anonymous where he receives support from "a higher power" and other people who have experienced victory with their alcoholism. The moral and spiritual support from Alcoholics Anonymous is without equal, and many people who follow their program faithfully return to active and useful lives in their communities.

Also of high value in helping the alcoholic recover are encouraging support from family members and hard work, which includes physical labor in an atmosphere free of alcohol and other addictive substances such as cigarettes. Most alcoholics are also addicted to nicotine. Successfully giving up smoking can help reinforce the decision to give up alcohol. Aerobic exercise, like jogging, walking or hard physical labor, is of great help in preventing the return to alcohol. Avoiding sugar and eating regular meals of vitamin rich foods, can help the body resist imbalances in blood sugar levels which may cause recovered alcoholics to crave alcohol. Supplements of vitamins, especially B vitamins, can help correct some of the physical imbalances caused by alcoholism. Large, 500 mg., doses of niacin taken at mealtimes under a doctor's supervision may help reduce craving for alcohol.

All efforts to treat alcoholism should be carried on with the support of competent physicians, concerned relatives and friends and pastoral care.

## Allergy Relief

Common allergies which produce wheezing, sneezing or difficult breathing are often caused by pollen or house dust. If you suffer from allergies, there are several natural methods of reducing your susceptibility.

1. Give your house a good vacuuming, but not by a person who suffers from allergies, since vacuuming stirs up a lot of dust. The best way to vacuum your house is to use a built-into-the-wall vacuuming system to keep the dust from the bag from getting stirred up into the living areas of the house.

When you vacuum, be sure to vacuum all of the bedding, including your mattresses. One of the most frequent causes of allergies from household dust is the presence of the microscopic remains of small mites, which lived in mattresses and pillows. A good vacuuming of mattresses, particularly in the areas where the head, neck and shoulders rest, will greatly reduce the number of mite remains in the bedding. Mites are especially concentrated in these areas, because they live on remains of skin and dandruff which flake off of people as they sleep.

When cleaning your house, vacuum far down into your ventilation pipes if you have forced-air heating or cooling; then vacuum the pipes coming out of your furnace. If you can afford it, professional cleaning companies can do a very good job of thoroughly cleaning and disinfecting your ventilation system.

2. Keep the humidity in your house relatively high in the dry months of the year like late fall and winter. A humidifier attached to your furnace is excellent for this.

3. If you suffer from allergies caused by pollen such as pine pollen in the spring and ragweed pollen in the summer and fall, you can often find relief by staying indoors and installing an electronic air filter in your air-conditioning system. If you don't have an electronic filter or if you can't afford one, be sure to change your regular filters frequently.

4. If you don't get significant relief from allergy symptoms caused by airborn particles like house dust and pollen by trying to avoid them, you may be able to reduce your symptoms by taking vitamin C. In one study, people who took 500 milligrams of vitamin C supplements

daily experienced less than half the number of allergy symptoms after taking vitamin C than they did before. Caution: If you take vitamin C, be very careful about taking exceptionally large doses of more than 500 milligrams per day. Also, to avoid stomach irritation, take vitamin supplements after meals. Be sure to check with your doctor for his advice.

### Alzheimer's Disease

Alzheimer's disease is a senile deterioration of the mind which usually results in death within a few months or years after the first symptoms become evident. Memory loss is one of the chief symptoms of Alzheimer's disease, but an accurate diagnosis should be made by a competent physician, since some memory loss is normal as people age. No one knows the cause of Alzheimer's disease. Some physicians suspect a slow acting virus or viral particle which attacks the brain. Some physicians think an autoimmune reaction to antigens in cigarette smoke may be one cause of the disease, because smokers are four times more likely to get the disease than non-smokers.

There is no cure for Alzheimer's disease, which may be fatal within a year or two, but the vitamin choline is reported in one study to slightly slow down the irreversible brain deterioration or at least to improve memory somewhat in the sufferers of this disease.

Autopsies of Alzheimer victims have revealed higher than normal levels of aluminum in the brain tissue.

Theoretically, preventing the accumulation of aluminum in elderly people may slow or prevent the development of the disease, but scientific studies haven't been completed to prove or disprove this theory. Avoiding foods containing aluminum or drinking three glasses of skim milk per day or taking fluoride supplements may prevent the accumulation of aluminum in the brain in Alzheimer victims, according to some researchers

See also: **Senility**

## Anemia

Anemia is a low level of red blood cells. It can be caused by many things, including serious diseases. Any symptoms of anemia should be brought to the attention of a competent physician. Anemia often occurs in women who have heavy menstrual flow.

Anemia which is not caused by serious disease often can be treated successfully with moderate supplements of iron, copper or multi-vitamin/ mineral supplements. Large doses of vitamin supplements should not be taken immediately before seeing a physician, because they might interfere with tests to spot serious conditions, like pernicious anemia which may be caused by an inability to absorb vitamin B12.

Pernicious anemia is treated successfully with injections of B12.

### Anorexia Nervosa

Anorexia Nervosa is a disorder of the appetite in which dieters, usually women, lose their appetite to such a great extent that they starve their bodies. People with this illness are often obsessed with being slim, and they come to look upon every food with distaste. One similar disorder is Bulimia, where a dieter will often eat a meal to keep up appearances and then go to a restroom and stick a finger down the throat to vomit up the stomach contents before they are absorbed by the body.

Psychiatrists have long considered Anorexia Nervosa to be a mental illness. Recent research indicates that, regardless of the causes which initially triggered the illness and for which psychotherapy may be beneficial, a key factor in the illness is a change in levels of the hormone vasopressin in the body. Vasopressin regulates blood pressure and, to a certain extent, appetite. When people become obsessed with dieting, their bodies often go through actual biochemical changes related to vasopressin levels and other factors. Then, it becomes difficult for them to get back to normal on their own.

Now, there's hope for people with Anorexia Nervosa. In recent studies, zinc supplements were quite successful in helping victims regain their appetites and recover. A study shows that more than 80% of Anorexia patients made a good recovery after taking zinc supplements. After treatment, they regained much of the weight they had lost and experienced a return to psychological balance in their attitudes toward eating.

Apparently, levels of zinc in the body often reach very low levels in crash dieting, and, because of the loss of this mineral, people may lose their senses of smell and taste and find that food is unappetizing. Zinc supplements help people to regain their senses of taste and smell and to enjoy eating once again. The recommended daily dietary allowance (RDA) for zinc is 15 milligrams per day for adults. Massive doses of zinc can cause serious side effects, but two or three times the RDA may be safely taken under a physician's care for a few weeks.

In addition to zinc, other vitamin and mineral supplements may be helpful in combating Anorexia Nervosa, because vitamins and minerals have a general stimulating effect on the entire body, including appetite. In some cases, loss of appetite may be caused by an overdose of calcium or deficiency of thiamine (vitamin B1), pantothenic acid, (vitamin B5), vitamin B12, biotin, phosphorus or zinc. Loss of appetite is also a common side effect of many prescription drugs, including diuretics (blood pressure lowering drugs), tranquilizers, antidepressants, anti-inflammatory drugs, antihistamines and sleeping aids.

Anorexia Nervosa has also been successfully treated by a prescription drug — Cyproheptadine. Anyone interested in treating Anorexia Nervosa with vitamins, minerals or prescription drugs should do it only under a doctor's care and advice, which may include counseling to help understand the psychological factors which may have precipitated the illness.

## Appendicitis

Appendicitis is an inflammation of the appendix of the large intestine. When it becomes infected, it may have to be removed by surgery. Although an appendectomy is a fairly routine operation, no surgical procedure is without a certain amount of danger to the patient.

The typical American low-fiber diet has been implicated as a major cause of appendicitis. Appendectomies are the most frequently performed abdominal emergency operations in the United States today (some 300,000 per year), while appendicitis is almost unknown among populations with a high-fiber content in their diets.

The vermiform (meaning wormlike) appendix is a part of the body with no obvious use, but it plays a part, like tonsils, in the body's immune system. It may help to prevent certain intestinal diseases, so the wisdom of routinely removing it during other abdominal surgery is questionable. It is an appendage to the large intestine, and it may be less than an inch long or as long as nine inches. Its average length is about three inches. The appendix shares the fecal contents of a cul-de-sac pouch called the cecum, which forms the first part of the colon. Normally, any fecal material flowing into the appendix is dumped right back into the cecum. But, if the opening to the appendix should become blocked by a stony concretion that may form around a piece of fecal material, inflammation of the appendix, or appendicitis, results. Western physicians say that surgery to remove the inflamed organ must be performed immediately when this happens or fatal peritonitis may result. Peritonitis is infection in the abdominal cavity caused by perforation and a resultant spreading of liquid feces throughout the abdomen. However, mainland Chinese physicians claim that they have successfully treated certain cases of appendicitis with laxatives instead of surgery. Our doctors warn that laxatives can cause an inflamed appendix to burst with fatal complications

Before about 1880, appendicitis was a rare condition. Slowly, thereafter, it began to increase in incidence in Britain and the United

States. In the 1920's, a distinguished British physician, Dr. Arthur Rendle Short, suggested that the main cause of appendicitis was the removal of much of the cellulose content of food. (The cellulose content of food is what we now know as dietary fiber.) He found that appendicitis was nearly ten times more common among schoolboys attending posh private schools, who had a steady diet of white bread, cakes and pastries, than it was among orphans who were fed much coarser bread.

Today's epidemiological evidence the world over shows without a doubt that appendicitis is most prevalent in communities consuming a low-fiber diet and is rare or unknown in communities on a high-fiber and low-sugar diet. Studies from various African countries (Ghana, Kenya, Natal, Nigeria, Rhodesia, South Africa, Sudan, Uganda, Zaire) show that appendicitis is still very rare throughout rural Africa but is becoming increasingly common among urban Africans who have adopted a typically western low-fiber diet.

Appendicitis can also increase or decrease within a few months of adopting new eating patterns. During World War II, for example, some Sudanese troops in North Africa were fed British Army rations (a change for them from a high to a low-fiber diet), and appendicitis became prevalent among them. Examples are also cited of a decreased incidence of appendicitis during war time when there was, of necessity in many countries, a return to less sophisticated, unprocessed foods. For example, in Switzerland during World War II, the incidence of appendicitis dropped when the Swiss ate less refined bread, consumed more vegetables, and cut their consumption of refined carbohydrates such as sugar.

Almost all cases of appendicitis can be prevented by eating a diet which is high in dietary fiber, like bran. A good way to start the day is with a bran cereal or a whole grain cereal. Lunch should include whole grain breads or soup laced with bran, as well as fresh fruits or vegetables. Supper could include fresh vegetables, such as corn which is high in dietary fiber, as well as other whole grain products like brown rice. Desserts can be made with bran or whole wheat flour. It's easy to substitute or add bran to many dessert recipes.

**Appetite, Loss of:** see **Anorexia Nervosa**

**Arteries , Hardening of:** see **Coronary Heart Disease**

**Arthritis**

Usually doctors will recommend rest, an

exercise program and thermal (heat) treatments to relieve arthritis naturally. Patients also are reminded to eat a well-balanced diet, maintain good posture and follow all the therapy prescribed by the doctor.

Rest - Especially during flare-ups, plenty of rest should be taken. People with arthritis should stop activities that cause severe pain, and they should never become completely exhausted. Tiredness and severe fatigue often contribute to arthritis, and naps may become part of the daily routine. A balance between rest and activity is needed to prevent inflammation and further damage to affected joints.

Exercise - A proper balance of rest and exercise helps to control arthritis. Exercise is needed to keep joints flexible, restore freedom of movement, improve circulation, and increase mobility. Specific exercise programs often are required to keep muscles and tendons strong and healthy, preventing further stress on joints.

Each person should consult a physician and often a physical therapist about an individual exercise program based on his or her needs. Different joints require different types and amounts of exercise to maintain the full range of motion. Isometric exercises are often advised. Isometrics are exercises that involve muscle contractions while the joints remain in place, like squeezing the hand against a fixed object.

Good general exercises are walking, hiking, swimming and bicycling. Hard sports should be avoided. All exercise should be preceded by warm-up to relax the muscles and prevent injuries.

Movements should be slow and gentle, never jarring the joints. The popular exercise motto "no pain, no gain" is NOT true for people who have arthritis. Arthritis sufferers should NEVER exercise to, or beyond, the point of pain.

Regular, doctor-approved exercise should be done at least 15 minutes a day, 5 to 7 days a week. During flare-ups when joints are very swollen, red and tender to the touch, exercises should be alternated with periods of rest, or exercising should be discontinued.

Exercising in water, known as hydrotherapy, sometimes is recommended because water helps support the joints during exercising. This allows the person to exercise all major muscle groups without putting stress on the affected joints. The Arthritis Foundation, in cooperation with the YMCA's and YWCA's, offers "exercising in the water" or "warm water" programs especially for sensitive joints.

Thermal Therapy - Heat is an excellent way to relieve pain, relax muscles, increase joint mobility and decrease joint and tissue inflammation. A hot shower or bath in the morning can loosen stiffness which invades joints during sleep or limber up stiff joints before exercising.

There are numerous ways to apply heat such as hot packs, heat lamps, electric pads, whirlpools, hot springs, saunas and warm paraffin wax treatments. Moist heat is usually preferable to dry heat. Sustaining comfortable heat levels for a longer period of time is better than applying heat that is too hot. Be careful to ensure that skin is protected from burns.

You can make excellent hot packs by soaking towels in hot water, then covering them with plastic wrap to hold the heat for as long as possible.

Hot wax treatments use melted paraffin applied to the affected joints. The best way to melt the paraffin is in an electric deep fat fryer, but the top of a double boiler can also be used. Wax maintains the heat on your body for long periods of time, but it can be messy or dangerous and should not be used if there are open cuts. If you and your doctor think that you are capable of handling paraffin wax, take precautions. Use a candy thermometer and don't heat the paraffin above 110°F. Keep a fire extinguisher handy and practice putting a lid on the double boiler with a long handled fork in case the paraffin catches on fire. Wax is easiest to use on small joints such as the hands, wrists, or feet.

Arthritis symptoms sometimes respond better to cold treatments with the aid of compresses or ice packs which can reduce inflammation. Alternating warm and cold sources on the affected area is known to help some arthritic sufferers.

Thermal therapy is not a wonder cure for arthritis. It is a way of reducing pain and inflammation. This helps arthritis sufferers to participate in everyday activities.

Joint Protection - Many people can relieve symptoms by learning to use joints carefully and relieving extra pressure on inflamed areas. Canes, walkers, and crutches can reduce the amount of body weight placed on joints. Splints or braces may be used to hold joints in position and protect them. Good posture can protect joints and prevent further damage.

Shoes should be purchased with extra care, because the feet support the body's weight. High heels should be avoided. They don't distribute body weight evenly, and they cause awkward walking. Low-heeled shoes that provide solid support, lots of room for the toes to move, a snug heel and cushioning make it easier to walk with correct posture and protect the joints.

Do everyday activities in a way that will least likely affect the arthritic joints. For example, rather than lifting large items, slide them across the floor. Use purses or pocketbooks with shoulder straps rather than carrying all the weight with the fingers and wrist. Push suitcases on wheels rather than carrying them. When trying to tackle everyday situations, consider your joints first — and you can protect them from unnecessary stress and further damage.

Diet and Nutrition For Arthritis - Nutrition plays an important role in preventing many illnesses, but a specific diet has never been proven to always help control any form of arthritis except gout. Arthritis sufferers should eat a well-balanced diet to consume the government recommended daily allowance (RDA's) of vitamins and minerals to maintain stamina and health.

Of course, obesity places more strain on inflamed joints. A weight reduction diet may be recommended by doctors to reduce pressure on the joints.

Some people, including a number of

physicians, claim that a diet largely composed of unsalted rice, excluding dairy products, wheat, meat, except fish, and all processed foods, is helpful for some cases of arthritis, particularly in cases of rheumatoid arthritis. No one has made controlled studies that support testimonials from people who claim to have been helped by such a diet.

Such a diet theoretically could be helpful to some people, even though this is unproven. Researchers recently have discovered anti-inflammatory properties in fish oil. Allergic reactions by some people to certain foods could possibly cause arthritis symptoms. The Arthritis Foundation recommends that if you suspect a certain food is aggravating your arthritis, try avoiding it for at least two weeks; then see if it makes a difference.

A diet low in cholesterol, fat and sodium could improve a person's physical well-being. It might help people who suffer from obesity, heart disease, high blood pressure, or other degenerative diseases associated with eating excessive amounts of high-fat or high-sodium foods. If this diet, or any other diet, helps a person lose excess weight, it may help relieve arthritis symptoms by reducing strain on weight-bearing joints.

There are two dangers to avoid if you go on

such a diet. Rice is a very healthful food, but it is not complete. You need vitamins, minerals and protein from vegetables, fruit and animal protein like fish. Make sure your doctor agrees that any diet you go on is well-balanced. Also, don't put all your faith in an unproven diet and neglect proven treatments.

Avoiding Quack Cures - Since arthritis is a "flare-up" kind of disease, many people will attribute sudden relief to the latest thing they have taken or tried. It is important to remember that, so far, no medical cure exists for arthritis.

Remissions have caused people to claim that everything from copper bracelets to pineapples can cure arthritis. For every dollar spent in arthritis research, $25.00 will be spent on expensive, unproven remedies.

Strange tales of "how I cured my arthritis" are often caused by the "placebo effect". A "placebo" is a harmless substance given to a patient. The patient is told that it will cure her disease — and because the patient really wants to be cured, or believes that she will be cured, it works!

The Arthritis Foundation used to call all "cures" that were not medically accepted, "quack cures." But now the Arthritis Foundation is being more cautious and refers to them as "unproven" remedies. These "cures" have not been medically proven to cure arthritis, and many of them can even be very harmful. But since cures for other diseases have been found in unusual places, like penicillin from mold, perhaps researchers will discover the long awaited cure for arthritis in an unusual remedy. Until then, unproven cures may be harmful and are not recommended.

"Unproven cures" fall into these four categories: drugs and medications, devices, publicized clinics, and nutrition ideas. To avoid these unproven remedies, arthritis sufferers should be leery of remedies that contain "secret" ingredients, remedies advertised for all types of arthritis, anything advertised as a "cure" for arthritis, and remedies that rely only on the claims of everyday people but have no valid, controlled medical or scientific research supporting them.

<u>Vitamins</u> <u>and</u> <u>Minerals</u> <u>for</u> <u>Arthritis</u> - Since aspirin causes vitamin C to be eliminated from the body, people taking large doses of aspirin (for arthritis) may benefit from vitamin C supplements.

Menopausal arthritis may be reduced with pyridoxine (vitamin B6) supplements.

Some arthritis sufferers claim that pantothenic acid (vitamin B5) is effective in reducing pain. A number of British physicians think that pantothenic acid supplements can prevent the development of rheumatoid arthritis and even osteoarthritis in many people. Long-term, controlled studies will be necessary to verify this claim.

## Backache

If you have a backache, particularly a serious one, you should see a doctor to make sure it's not a symptom of a serious disease. If the backache is a result of strain, there are simple steps you can take to reduce pain and speed recovery.

First, lie down and give your back muscles a chance to relax so that the painful spasm can go away. Applications of cold compresses may be helpful. Later on, after the immediate spasm has passed, applications of heat to the area of pain may help to loosen up muscles. Soothing ointments which are advertised to help relieve back pain or increase blood flow may also be helpful once the initial spasm has passed. Many doctors also prescribe aspirin to help reduce pain and inflammation during the recovery period.

Once recovery has taken place, there are several steps you can take to reduce the chances of future injury. Most back pain occurs because the muscles in the lower back, which help support the spine, are weak from lack of use. Simple exercises which don't strain the back are helpful in building up the strength of these muscles.

1. The best gentle back exercise is to lie flat on your back in bed and gradually increase the tension in your abdominal muscles. Next, alternately flatten and then slightly bow your back as you're lying on the bed.

2. If you're in fairly good shape, this exercise can help. Stand erect with feet spread apart and slowly bend from the waist until you touch your toes or come close to them. Then, slowly come back to an erect position. With this exercise, the emphasis is on the word "slowly". Sudden movements may cause the very back strain you're trying to guard against. After you've done this exercise for a few days, you can increase the number of repetitions periodically from 5 to 10 to 20 to 30 or more. At this point, your muscles will have gotten stronger so you won't be as likely to strain your back in the future.

3. You can also do sit-up exercises to help strengthen the abdominal muscles which help promote good posture. Lie down on the floor with your back flat on the floor and your knees elevated so that your legs slope up at a 45 degree angle. Put your hands on your chest and slowly

rise to a sitting position. If this exercise causes strain, just raise your head and shoulders off the ground until this exercise has helped you to get into better shape. At that point, try to do a full sit-up. Again, always sit up with the knees elevated so that the leg forms a 45 degree angle. This elevation of the knees is quite helpful in preventing back strain while doing the exercise.

4. Good posture is important in preventing back strain. Try to lift objects, using your legs by bending your knees to reach them instead of bending from the back. Avoid sudden movements which twist the body. Be sure to sit erect with your back not slumped over. When you're working while standing, work at a comfortable level so that you don't have to bend over to reach your work.

5. When you're sleeping, a soft mattress is usually the worst thing for back support. If possible, buy a very firm mattress or put a sheet of plywood between your mattress and box springs to give your body extra support.

6. Many cases of back pain occur because people have flat feet or because one leg is shorter than the other. If you have one leg that is shorter than the other, a special shoe can help even out the difference and balance out the forces on your backbone while you're standing. If you have flat feet or poor arches, arch

supports can help even out tensions which are transmitted through the leg to the backbone.

If you conscientiously follow all the above advice, you can minimize the chance of suffering common backaches if there is not a serious underlying disease which is causing the problem.

Many people with backaches or other aches and pains pay frequent visits to chiropractors. Chiropractic treatment can hardly be called a natural way of dealing with physical problems, because it involves taking x-rays and manipulating the spine by a skilled practitioner. Some medical doctors claim that there is no value to chiropractic treatment and that most chiropractors are quacks. Some chiropractors respond that medical doctors don't care about the total well-being of their patients and often deal with them in a detached, impersonal manner.

I once asked a wise medical doctor what he thought of chiropractic treatment, and he told me that at least one-half of what physicians and other healers do is give the patient assurance that he's going to get better because of a particular type of treatment. Later, the patient often will get better, regardless of whether the treatment itself helped him.

This "placebo" effect is responsible for

much of the healing that takes place regardless of what sort of treatment is used or what sort of practitioner used the treatment. According to my friend, the medical doctor, most chiropractors excel in the area of giving the patient confidence that he will get better because of their treatment.

When the "placebo" effect is combined with the body's own God-given ability to heal itself, the work of chiropractors, if they are sincerely interested in the welfare of their patients and if they are careful not to injure the spine, may sometimes surpass that of standard medical treatment.

Is there any benefit to chiropractic treatment in addition to the helpful psychological aspects? One scientific study which attempted to answer this question showed that patients who were treated for lower back pain through typical chiropractic manipulations experience more relief from pain than other patients who were treated in a different way as a control population. Unfortunately, this study showed the total healing time of the patients treated with chiropractic manipulation was greater than the patients in the control group.

There are not many good scientific studies on the effectiveness of chiropractic treatment. On the positive side, it seems to make some people feel better, and many people testify to this. On the negative side, many medical doctors point out that it is quite possible to seriously injure the spine by manipulation and to cause injury to other parts of the body. One recent study by an M.D. showed that many elderly people experienced strokes soon after receiving chiropractic manipulation in the neck area. Medical doctors caution that spinal manipulation is less dangerous when it is performed in the lower back than when it is performed in the neck or upper back.

**Bad Breath**

Bad breath frequently is caused by eating sugary foods, which allows large numbers of bacteria to grow in the mouth. Eliminating sugary foods from the diet, using dental floss and brushing the tongue as well as the teeth with the toothbrush may be helpful. In addition, periodically sterilizing toothbrushes, by dipping them into a diluted solution of hydrogen peroxide and then rinsing well with water may help to prevent excess bacteria from growing in the mouth.

Bad breath is also often caused by constipation. With constipation, bacteria cause the fecal mass in the intestines to ferment and produce noxious smelling gases which are then absorbed into the bloodstream and ventilated through the lungs. If bad breath is caused by constipation, it can be treated by eating plenty of dietary fiber like bran, substituting whole grain products for white flour or sugar-containing foods and avoiding a diet which leads to constipation.

**Baldness**

Baldness usually occurs through a hereditary gene which is expressed most noticeably in males, although females may exhibit a small degree of hair loss late in life. There are certain remedies for baldness, but they usually involve the application of drugs which have side effects. Estrogen creams rubbed on the head have been shown to reduce hair loss, but they have also caused feminizing side effects, such as enlargement of the breasts in many men who have used them.

A new prescription drug, Minoxidil®, has been shown to greatly reduce hair loss, but it can cause side effects in people who use it.

Natural means of avoiding hereditary baldness are less successful. The vitamins inositol and biotin taken internally or rubbed on the scalp in the form of ointments or shampoos may slightly reduce hair loss, but successful prevention of hair loss by using them is quite limited.

See also: **Hair Loss.**

**Birth Defects**

The chance of birth defects can be greatly decreased if pregnant women take certain precautions.

1. Don't smoke. Smoking is proven to increase birth defects.

2. Don't drink alcohol. The "fetal alcohol syndrome" is a form of retardation which is proven to be caused by drinking alcohol, especially excessive amounts of alcohol, during pregnancy.

3. Be careful in taking prescription drugs. Many drugs have been proven to increase the incidence of birth defects in pregnant women who take them. Consult carefully with your doctor about the chance of birth defects before taking any prescription drug, and only take the drug if it is proven not to cause birth defects or if the benefits of taking the drug far outweigh the risk to the unborn child.

4. Take vitamin supplements. Women who have had children with birth defects and who are at greater statistical risk for having birth defects in future offspring have been greatly

helped by taking vitamin supplements, including supplements of folic acid. As a matter of fact, many obstetricians recommend that pregnant women take regular multi-vitamin supplements to prevent birth defects and to help the overall health of the mother and the development of the baby.

### Bladder Infections

Bladder infections usually occur because of the migration of bacteria from the genital area up through the urethra to the bladder. They are much more of a problem for women than for men, because urethras in women are much shorter, and it's easier for bacteria to make a short trip than a long trip.

Antibiotics, especially sulfa drugs, can clear up most bladder infections quickly if taken soon after symptoms appear.

The first method of preventing bacterial infections is to bathe frequently, using showers instead of tub baths. Sitting in a tub bath can wash bacteria from the genital area well up into the urethra in just a few minutes. It's also important for men and women to wipe from front to back rather from back to front after elimination.

Many bladder infections are related to lack

of washing by either partner before intercourse. It's also extremely important to completely void the bladder and to wash the genital area within a few minutes after intercourse. This last tip is probably as important as all of the other tips combined.

### Blindness (Night Blindness)

Loss of vision in near darkness is an early symptom of vitamin A deficiency. Vitamin A deficiency can be prevented by regularly eating yellow vegetables like carrots.

### Blood Clots

Many older people have a tendency for blood clots to form in the legs and other parts of the body. Blood clots can be life-threatening if they block circulation, or if they become dislodged and travel to the lungs or brain where they may cause a stroke.

Blood clots are less likely to form when people are active. Bedridden patients, like those recovering from surgery, should be encouraged to get up and walk. Patients who cannot walk should be encouraged to move around in bed or be turned frequently.

Vitamin E is reported to have an

anticoagulant (anti-clotting) effect. It has been used to treat people with poor leg circulation, called intermittent claudication. People with intermittent claudication have a tendency to have leg cramps, experience pain when walking, and form blood clots in the legs.

Niacin (vitamin B3) is a vasodilator (blood-vessel enlarger). It may improve circulation in the elderly and thus keep legs and arms from falling asleep. It may also help to prevent blood clots from forming. The overall effectiveness of this use is unknown, and it may vary from person to person.

Niacin or vitamin E should only be used under the advice of a physician. Caution should be used in taking large doses which can cause serious side effects. Caution should also be used in taking supplements of the vitamin pantothenic acid (vitamin B5). Pantothenic acid supplements may reduce the effectiveness of anticoagulant drugs (blood thinners) which are used to prevent blood from clotting.

### Blood Pressure, High

High blood pressure is one of modern society's worst enemies. An estimated 60 million Americans have some form of hypertension ( the medical term for high blood pressure). Although it is rarely listed on death certificates as the cause of death, high blood pressure, if left untreated, can lead to numerous other causes of death. Strokes, heart attacks, and kidney failure are major examples of the devastation of this elusive illness.

In most, but not all cases, high blood pressure can be lowered without prescription drugs. For example, in one recent university test, 85.3% of patients with high blood pressure were able to quit taking medication. Even without drugs, their blood pressures remained lower than when they were on drugs. The hundreds of people in the study also found that their blood cholesterol levels dropped 26%. The doctor in charge of the program said, "You lose your tiredness. You feel much more active. You have a general feeling of well being." The patients learned the health secrets described below and began making changes in their eating and exercise habits.

## Common Causes of High Blood Pressure

*Salt* - Studies of different nations around the world show that high blood pressure is a problem only in societies where people eat a lot of sodium, usually in the form of salt. High blood pressure rates are in direct proportion to the amount of salt consumed. The more salt that a particular society consumes, the greater the number of cases of severe high blood pressure.

The average American eats five to ten grams of sodium per day, but most people only need one tenth that amount. However, there are exceptions: hard manual labor, pregnancy and breast feeding may increase the need for sodium to as much as 2 grams per day.

Most people will question whether they really consume one-third to one-fifth of an ounce of salt per day, but processed foods that Americans eat are usually filled with salt. Any food that comes in a can, a frozen package or a box is likely to have salt added as a preservative or flavor enhancer.

Many scientific studies show that reducing salt intake will lower blood pressure in most people by a significant amount. Getting salt intake down into the range of 500 mg. of salt per day helps the most. Reducing salt intake lowers blood pressure dramatically in some people who have a tendency toward high blood pressure; thus, the benefits of reduced salt consumption are greater for people who need the benefits the most, those with life and health-threatening high blood pressure.

*Vitamins Which Affect Blood Pressure* - An overdose of vitamin D from either excessive exposure to the sun, which acts on the skin to help produce Vitamin D, or from taking high doses of vitamin D supplements can lead to high blood pressure. Vitamin E, in doses larger than the RDA, can cause high blood pressure.

Choline supplements are reported to help control blood pressure. In one study, one-third of a group of patients with high blood pressure had their blood pressure return to normal after receiving choline supplements. When the supplements were discontinued, their blood pressure rose once again. However, additional studies are needed to confirm that choline alone was responsible.

*Cadmium and Lead* - Cadmium is a "heavy metal" which may be found in small trace amounts in water supplies in the United States and in other countries. The cause-and-effect relationship between high levels of cadmium and high blood pressure exists as it does with salt. Studies indicate that other heavy metals, like lead, may also contribute to high blood pressure. Your local water authority may be able to tell you if your water supply has higher than average concentrations of cadmium or lead. If it does, certified pure bottled water would be a good alternative.

*Drugs* - Caffeine, diet pills and many prescription and over-the-counter drugs can raise blood pressure significantly. Caffeine is found in most "cola" and "pepper" drinks, coffee, tea and chocolate. Your pharmacist or your doctor can tell you if any prescription drugs you are taking can raise blood pressure. Also, be sure to read the warnings listed on any non-prescription medicines you may buy.

*Pollution* - Smog, smoking tobacco or breathing tobacco smoke has a significant effect in raising blood pressure.

We are all familiar with such pollution as smog, but do you know that excessive noise pollution raises blood pressure? It's true. Studies have shown that people who work in noisy environments have lower blood pressures after there is a significant reduction of noise in their work areas.

*Lack of Exercise* - Many studies indicate that various types of exercise help to control high blood pressure. Exercise which increases the strength of the heart may help to prevent or lower high blood pressure. Aerobic exercise, such as jogging, swimming, walking and playing tennis, can lower blood pressure. Also, surprisingly, isometric exercises which involve little body movement, are useful as relaxation training to reduce blood pressure.

Before starting an exercise program consult a physician and follow a recommended plan.

Remember to slowly increase the intensity and duration of exercise. Don't overdo it in the beginning. Watch for body signals, such as sharp pains and cramps, that tell you when you're doing too much. Walking is usually recommended by doctors as the best beginning exercise for people who are out of shape.

*Diets High In Fat* - Americans now consume almost 40% of their total calories from fat. Cutting fat intake levels in half can have a dramatic effect in reducing many cases of high blood pressure. A recent study by the U.S. Department of Agriculture found that eating less saturated fat could bring blood pressure down even in the absence of taking other beneficial measures. Replacing saturated fats, which are found in meat and shortening, with vegetable oil or fish oil may also help reduce high blood pressure. Remember, fats are present not only in butter, oil and margarine, but also in fried foods, chips, creamed sauces, mayonaise, pastries, cheese, to name a few. Learn to read labels on cans and packages, looking for the fat content listed.

*Alcohol* - Excessive alcohol drinking is a major cause of high blood pressure. In fact, it's the #1 villain among people who drink more than one ounce of alcohol (2 drinks) per day. Alcohol makes blood pressure skyrocket as it damages the liver and kidneys and causes fluid build-up.

### Natural Protection Against High Blood Pressure

*Potassium* - There is evidence that potassium may help protect against high blood pressure. Part of the evidence, however, is clouded by the fact that societies which have high levels of salt consumption also have low levels of potassium consumption and vice versa.

It certainly wouldn't hurt most people to start eating more foods like bananas and citrus fruits, especially grapefruit, which are relatively high in potassium. Potassium supplements can be considered but should not be used by people who have kidney disease or who are taking a prescription diuretic that is potassium-sparing.

*Calcium* - A recent study indicates that people with high blood pressure consume 20% - 25% less calcium than people who don't have high blood pressure. Calcium is found in water and certain foods. The RDA of calcium is 800 -

1200 mg. per day for adult males and females. Supplementation above this level isn't usually necessary.

*Magnesium* - A recent study by Dr. Burton M. Altura links low magnesium levels to high blood pressure. He believes that if the level of magnesium is too low, the calcium level becomes too high and the blood vessels contract, causing high blood pressure. In a separate study by Cornell University, Dr. Lawrence Resnick discovered that people with high blood pressure tend to have low magnesium in their red blood cells. Futhermore, Resnick claims that the patients who have normal blood pressure have higher magnesium levels.

Other studies show that people have lower blood pressure if their water supplies have high concentrations of magnesium. Magnesium often is found with calcium in drinking water and in mineral supplements like Dolomite.

*False High Blood Pressure* - Hardening of the arteries in the elderly may cause high, inaccurate blood pressure readings, Dr. Frank H. Messerli, a blood pressure specialist reported in the New England Journal of Medicine.

Messerli discovered that people over 65 with hardened arteries had higher blood pressure when monitored with a blood pressure cuff than their true blood pressure taken using a needle inside the arteries. Hardened arteries are caused by fatty or calcium deposits in the arteries. (See also Coronary Heart Disease.)

Another kind of false high blood pressure is often called the "white coat syndrome". Many people, up to 30%, are diagnosed as having high blood pressure because they are nervous when their blood pressure is taken at their doctor's office. Home blood pressure readings, or 24-hour monitoring, can help give doctors a better picture of a patient's true blood pressure.

### Breast Enlargement

Breast enlargement is something that may sometimes be desired in women but not in men. There are many devices and products on the market which claim to enlarge breasts in women, and there are many ads in mass market women's magazines for such products. All of these products have been successfully challenged by the government and have been proved to be of little value.

One type of product is an exerciser which a woman presses between her hands in front of her chest. This is said to increase the size and firmness of the pectoral muscles which run from the shoulder down to the breast. While there may be some effect of such exercise devices on the pectoral muscles, there is no effect on the actual breast tissue. As a matter of fact, heavy exercise may increase the production of androgenic or male-like hormones in women. This increase in androgenic hormones may actually lead to a decrease in breast size.

Another product is a cream which is claimed to contain estrogen or progesterone or some other similar compound. If a woman rubs this on her breast, she is supposed to see a gradual enlargement. Such claims are somewhat questionable, and the use of a product for a specific medical purpose is forbidden by law unless the product has been approved by the FDA for that purpose and is relatively free of harmful side effects.

Many of the advertisements for breast enlargement products for women show "before and after" pictures of women who claim that the product has helped enlarge their breasts. However, breast enlargement occurs in women for many reasons, some of which have little to do with the use of products which have claimed to produce breast enlargement.

Women who become pregnant usually see an enormous increase in breast size as they approach the end of their pregnancy. If women nurse after giving birth, this breast enlargement will be maintained or increased. Birth control pills also frequently cause an enlargement in the breasts because of the higher circulating levels of female hormones. Young women in their teenage years may see substantial increases in their breasts even after the period immediately following their first menses. For these reasons, advertised claims for breast enlargers are questionable, and advertising for such products is frequently challenged successfully by governmental authorities.

Men may experience unwanted breast enlargement for a number of reasons. Young men in puberty may experience a temporary enlargement or hardness under the nipple which usually disappears after a few months or years as the hormonal fluctuation of puberty becomes evened out. Older men may experience some enlargement in their breasts as male hormone levels drop off in strength with increasing years. Men also sometimes experience breast enlargement as a side effect of an estrogen cream. One such cream was promoted a few years ago for preventing hair loss in men, but a substantial number of men who used the cream soon noticed breast enlargement.

Desirable breast enlargement in young women can be promoted by eating a nutritious diet including an adequate number of calories, which may also promote overall weight gain and enlargement in other areas. Hormone supplements should only be taken to correct deficiencies, under a doctor's supervision.

Men can sometimes reduce the appearance of having enlarged breasts by overall weight reduction or by engaging in strenuous exercise which promotes the production of androgenic hormones and the development of firm, muscle tissue. Taking anabolic steroid hormones to increase masculine characteristics is not advised for most men because of serious side effects. Anabolic steroids should only be taken on a doctor's advice.

### Burn Treatment

Serious burns should be treated by a physician. Minor burns may be treated at home only if the epidermis, the outer layer of the skin, is burned without blistering.

One recently discovered home remedy for burns and minor wounds that's said to be remarkably effective is the application of a preparation advertised for treatment of hemorrhoids, which contains a yeast culture. A recent scientific study showed that the application of this cream had a remarkable healing affect on minor burns and wounds.

Many people feel that application of vitamin E is superficial and should not be used on serious second or third degree burns.

If it is necessary to bandage a burn, use a teflon coated bandage which won't stick to the wound. The removal of a bandage which has stuck to the skin can be a painful procedure. If sticking occurs, removal may be made easier by dabbing with a diluted hydrogen peroxide solution.

## Cancer

Cancer is an unrestrained growth of certain cells in the body. Some cancers are distributed throughout the body. Other cancers show up as tumors or clearly defined, rapidly growing masses of cells. Tumors can metastasize or spread from one distinct location in the body to other locations.

*Warning Signs of Cancer:*

1. Unusual bleeding or discharge.
2. A lump or thickening in any area.
3. A sore that does not heal.
4. A change in bowel or bladder habits.
5. Hoarseness or persistent cough.
6. Indigestion or difficulty in swallowing.

7. Change in the size, shape or appearance of a wart, mole or freckle.
8. Unexplained loss of weight.

Any of the above warning signals of cancer should be brought to the attention of a physcian immediately.

*What Causes Cancer*

There is no single cause of cancer, but there are many factors which can lead to its development. The first factor is a hereditary predisposition towards cancer. Because of their natural body constitution, some people are immune or more resistant to cancer than other people. A person whose constitution is not equipped to deal well with pre-cancerous changes will have a greater risk of getting cancer than other people.

The second major cause of cancer is radiation. Radiation from the sun is a proven contributor to skin cancer, particularly in fair skinned people. People who spend a lot of time at the beach or working out in the sun have much greater rates of skin cancer than others. The early discoverers of radioactive materials often suffered from cancer because of working closely with these materials. People who have had excessive exposure to x-rays, particularly from x-ray machines which were manufactured several years ago, are at a greater risk for cancer.

The third major factor leading to cancer is exposure to cancer-causing environmental substances (carcinogens). The first substance noticed by medical science was soot from chimneys. Over a century ago, small children in England who were used as chimney sweeps often came down with cancer of the testicles because of constant exposure to soot while climbing up and down chimneys.

Several decades ago, many scientists noticed that coal tar and coal tar products would cause cancer when applied to the skin of animals. Later, smoking and tar products from tobacco were proven to cause cancer.

Several decades ago, certain viruses were shown to cause cancer in animals. In recent years, viruses have been implicated in causing or contributing to the development of certain cancers in humans. The viral disease, Hepatitis B, is the major cause of liver cancer. Herpes Simplex virus has been implicated as a causative factor of cancer of the cervix in women. The Epstein-Barr virus can, under certain other environmental circumstances, lead to the development of Burkitt's Lymphoma. Viruses cause some, if not all, leukemias, but only in a small percentage of people who have been infected by the virus.

*Modern Treatment Methods for Cancer*

Surgery, when appropriate, is the most effective treatment for cancer. If a tumor can be completely removed by surgery before it spreads, there may be a low rate of recurrence. Successful surgery depends upon detecting cancer at an early stage when a tumor may be small and easy to remove. Later on in the illness, the tumor may be very large and difficult to remove, or it may have spread into other areas.

Radiation and chemotherapy are sometimes successful treatments, particularly against cancers of the blood cells. Much of modern medical science is devoted towards improving forms of chemotherapy and radiation treatment. In spite of this effort, a recent study indicated that there is very little difference in survival rates for most types of cancers today than there was thirty years ago. Tumors have certain characteristics which make the body's immunity system ineffective in attacking them. Tumors seem to secrete protective cocoons which interfere with the natural attacks of the body's immunity system. Tumors may also give off antigens through their protective cocoons, and the body is fooled into attacking these "distractions."

The most promising area of research in cancer treatment is strengthening the body's immunity system so that the body itself can naturally attack the cancer which is growing inside it. Some researchers have reported success with various vaccines for certain cancers, like melanoma. Vaccines to prevent virus-caused diseases may be effective in preventing cancer. A new vaccine for Hepatitis B could reduce the chance of getting liver cancer by 90%. Vaccines have been given to people after surgery for lung cancer, and the results are still being evaluated.

One promising new treatment involves the injection of monoclonal antibodies which are specifically activated to attack the patient's own cancer cells. Other hopeful areas of research involve the injection of substances such as interleukin-3, interferon and enzymes like streptokinase to help the body's own defenses.

For the latest development in medical treatment of cancer, call this number: 1-800-4-CANCER. This United States government sponsored information service can give you all the latest, up-to-date information.

## Health Tips To Help Prevent Cancer

There is no natural cure for cancer once it becomes established, but there are many things that we can do to help prevent cancer and to reduce our chances of getting it.

*Cancer Prevention Tip #1*

Avoid drinking or cooking with chlorinated water. Instead, use certified pure spring water. Lest anyone think this advice is unproven or unsound, I am reprinting substantial selected portions of a report published by the U.S. Environmental Protection Agency, Office of Research and Development, Health Effects Research Laboratory, Cincinnati, Ohio:

"REPORTS OF CASE CONTROL STUDY OF CANCER DEATHS IN FOUR SELECTED NEW YORK COUNTIES IN RELATION TO DRINKING WATER CHLORINATION by Michael Alavanja, Inge Goldstein and Mervyn Susser.

"Introduction

"Recent studies have pointed to the possibility that chlorination of drinking water may be related to gastrointestinal and urinary tract cancer mortality.

"To further examine this relationship we have done a retrospective case-control study for every female gastrointestinal and urinary tract cancer death in seven New York State counties for the years 1968-1970. Data was accumulated from county comprehensive water supply reports and from death certificates.

"Background information on related studies can be found in the literature review while details of our procedures are described in the methodology section.

"Methodology

"This study was confined to females because a majority of the female population list their occupation as housewife. Housewives, we assume, tend to consume a significantly larger proportion of their meals at home as compared to men of the same family. Moreover, occupational exposure to chemical carcinogens will tend to be less frequent in a female population, for even among employed women, few engage in activities which result in exposure to occupational carcinogens. Yet, to further insure thorough consideration of the possible confounding effects of occupational carcinogens the occupation of every liver and kidney case and control and a random sample of other gastrointestinal and urinary tract cases and control selected at random was extracted from inspection of actual death certificates. Data on occupation was analyzed by cross tabulation in an attempt to reveal any association between occupation and cancer in these counties.

"The seven New York State counties selected for study include Allegany, Cattaraugus, Chautauqua, Erie, Rensselaer, Schenectady, and St. Lawrence. These counties had a combined 1970 population of 1.81 million people and were chosen because they met the following criteria:

"1. The population of each county was served by at least three different types of water supply — chlorinated ground water, chlorinated surface water or nonchlorinated ground water. Well water usually provides a consistent source of water low in color and organic content. Surface water (water from rivers and lakes) is more frequently higher in color and organic content.

"2. For 15 years prior to the study period each county had a relatively stable population with regard to migration into and out of the county. This criterion is important because population stability, especially a low rate of immigration, will tend to insure long water-exposure histories.

"3. The population of each county did not experience a major change in the source, quality or distribution pattern of water for a period of fifteen years prior to the study dates.

"Detailed information concerning each of these criteria with regard to the seven selected counties is included in appendix I.

"The current study is limited by the dearth of chloroform concentration data for the water supplies of the seven selected counties. In order to overcome this limitation we are relying on the observations of Rook (18) that nonchlorinated waters have low chloroform concentration while chlorination of highly colored water produces the highest chloroform concentrations.

"The literature review presented at the beginning of this paper mentioned a number of known risk factors for liver and kidney cancer, and these constitute possible confounding variables. Among these were urban residence, alcoholism, analgesic abuse, hazardous occupation and tobacco use. Urban residence is a potential confounding variable because more urban residents drink chlorinated water than do rural residents. The urban factor is accounted for in the analysis by contrasting liver and kidney death rates by water type within the rural or urban residence category.

"Alcoholism, analgesic abuse, tobacco use and sex-hormone use could not be measured, estimated or controlled for in this study. Since, these variables are not known or suspected to be associated with water chlorination, except in so far as they have a different urban-rural distribution, they do not constitute a likely source of significant confounding error.

"Confounding error from employment in high risk industries was minimized by selecting only female gastrointestinal and urinary tract concerns. Estimation of the residual effect of this variable was made from the determination of occupation from death certificates.

"Results

"As mentioned previously, this study concerned itself solely with cases of gastrointestinal and urinary tract cancer among the female population of the 1.81 million people (1970) in the seven counties examined. The assumptions on which this selection was made — that women are less frequently exposed to the confounding effects of possible industrial carcinogens — was borne out when an examination of death certificates indicated that 85% of the cases and controls were housewives and the remaining 15% were involved in comparatively low cancer-risk occupations such as office work, teaching or nursing.

"Several conclusions can be drawn on the basis of a x2 analysis of the data accumulated for the female population studied. In all counties except for Erie it was found that when water type was not taken into account, urban dwellers were at equal risk with rural residents for gastrointestinal and urinary tract cancer mortality. When water type was taken into account it was found that those who lived in areas served by chlorinated water had a greater relative risk of dying of gastrointestinal and urinary tract cancer than those who lived in areas with nonchlorinated water supplies.

"When the data were broken down by urban/rural residence, the risk for urban females residing in areas supplied with chlorinated water was greater than for their counterparts served by nonchlorinated water.

"For rural residents the relationships become slightly more complex, but definitive statements cannot be made because of a relatively small number. It appears, however, that females who lived in rural areas served by chlorinated ground water had a slightly elevated risk of dying from gastrointestinal and urinary tract cancer than their counterparts receiving nonchlorinated water. In rural regions served by chlorinated surface water, however, female residents were at the same risk as those in rural areas receiving nonchlorinated water.

"An attempt was made to relate water color with cancer mortality but results were inconclusive because of a shortage of data — a problem we hope to rectify in a future study.

"Although scanty data also hindered development of any firm conclusions regarding relationships between water type and cancer of the kidney or liver specifically, it appears in the combined population of Erie and Schenectady counties (the two most populated counties) that **residents receiving chlorinated water had a higher risk of dying of these cancers than those persons serviced by nonchlorinated water.**" {my emphasis}

There are a number of other studies indicating that drinking chlorinated water may be an important factor contributing to the cause of several kinds of cancer.

*Cancer Prevention Tip #2*

Avoid using talcum powder in the genital areas. A study published a few years ago showed that women who use talcum powder in the genital areas or put it on sanitary napkins have a higher risk of ovarian cancer than those who don't use talcum powder. Talcum powder sold in foreign countries often contains asbestos,which is a proven cancer-causing substance. However, studies in the United States show that most brands of talcum powder sold here are asbestos-free or have a very low level of asbestos in them. This brings up the possibility that talcum powder itself, even if not contaminated with asbestos, may in some way lead to the development of cancer of the ovary.

### Cancer Prevention Tip #3

Avoid coffee. One study has shown that drinking coffee may lead to cancer of the pancreas. Fortunately for coffee drinkers, this study has not been confirmed by other researchers who have published papers indicating that this is not the case. Nevertheless, to be on the safe side, it would probably be best for people to skip their coffee drinking.

Also avoid decaffeinated coffee, except for decaffeinated coffee in which a water extraction process is used to remove the caffeine. Many manufacturers of decaffeinated coffee use a methylene chloride process, which can leave a residue of this cancer-causing chemical in the coffee.

*Cancer Prevention Tip #4*

Avoid asbestos. Asbestos is a proven, serious cancer-causing material. Cigarette smokers normally have up to 10 times the rate of lung cancer as non-smokers; but cigarette smokers who also are exposed to asbestos particles in the air have rates of lung cancer up to 100 times higher than the rest of the population. Asbestos is such a serious cancer-causing agent that manufacturers of asbestos products have been sued to the point of bankruptcy by many people who have become cancer victims after handling their products.

*Cancer Prevention Tip #5*

Avoid excessive exposure to the sun. Both common skin cancer and a deadly form of skin cancer called melanoma are related to overexposure to the sun. In recent years, fair skinned people have been spending more time at the beach and at swimming pools; and the rate of skin cancers has multiplied.

Sunshine need not be avoided entirely, but exposure to strong sunlight should be limited to no more than a few minutes without protection.

Additionally, people who swim, sunbathe or play sports out-of-doors, should wear protective clothing and use sunscreens which block most of the cancer-causing ultra-violet radiation from the sun.

*Cancer Prevention Tip #6*

Avoid fried foods. Fried foods are doubly bad as cancer-causing substances because they usually contain high percentages of fat, often of the saturated variety, and because frying itself can change the cooking fat into even more harmful cancer-causing substances. If a person feels it is necessary to fry food, it is better to use unprocessed cooking oil such as peanut oil instead of margarine, shortening, lard or cooking oils which have been chemically processed with the addition of hydrogen to make the oil more saturated than it was in its natural state.

*Cancer Prevention Tip #7*

Avoid processed foods which may have additives that can contribute to the development of cancer. It's good to avoid all artificially colored foods because they may contain certain food dyes which are suspected of causing cancer.    Read the labels of food products, especially processed meat products, to find out if they contain food dyes.

Most processed meats and most red meats have sodium nitrite added to act as a preservative and red coloring agent. Bacon, hot dogs and processed meats contains large amounts of this preservative. Sodium nitrite can react with other chemicals in the body to form cancer-forming substances called nitrosamines.

*Cancer Prevention Tip #8*

Avoid barrier forms of contraception, like condoms. A scientific study has shown that 71% of women who had breast cancer surgery had used barrier contraception, but only 34% of the control group had used this method. Estimates based on these studies indicate that 16% of all women who use barrier contraception and who do not have breast cancer will develop it at some point in the future, but only 3.4% of married women who don't use barrier contraception will develop breast cancer.

*Cancer Prevention Tip #9*

Eat foods rich in vitamin D, calcium,

molybdenum, and selenium, such as fish, whole grain foods, wheat germ and beans . Studies have shown high rates of cancer in people who have a low supply of these nutrients in their diet.

## Cancer Prevention Tip #10

Include lysine in your diet. A recent study commissioned by the Benjamin Franklin Literary and Medical Society showed that people who took supplements of the amino acid lysine had much lower rates of cancer than other people. Interestingly enough, there was no significant reduction in rates of cancer for people who took extra selenium, zinc, vitamin E, vitamin C, and vitamin A, even though taking supplements of these other nutrients has been suggested for cancer prevention. For people who prefer not to take supplements, skim milk is a good source of protein which contains lysine in relatively high amounts.

## Cancer Prevention Tip #11

Eat crunchy yellow and dark green leafy vegetables. Studies have shown that diets which are high in these vegetables are effective in reducing the incidence of certain cancers. Carrots, cauliflower, kale, spinach, broccoli and mustard greens all seem to help the body resist the development of cancer.

*Cancer Prevention Tip #12*

Reduce the amount of sodium in your diet and increase the amount of potassium. Population studies have shown that people living in areas of low sodium concentration in the water and high potassium concentration have low rates of cancer. The first step in cutting back on sodium is to stop salting your food or to replace the salt you were using with a type of "light" salt, which contains half potassium chloride and half sodium chloride.

Then, you should avoid most processed foods such as cured meat, ham, luncheon meat, and processed meals which are not advertised as being light in salt. Next, you should avoid salted snacks like potato chips, pretzels, pickles, nachos, T.V. dinners, canned foods, processed cheese and margarine, and bread containing salt.

After you've eliminated some of these gremlins from your diet, you should replace them with fresh fruits and fresh vegetables. These are all generally high in potassium and relatively low in sodium. Ideally, sodium and potassium should be in about a one-to-one ratio;

so that for every milligram of sodium in your diet you should also have a milligram of potassium. Most people on American diets consume 3 or 4 times as much sodium as potassium.

### Cancer Prevention Tip #13

Eat cereals and whole grain products. These foods contain dietary fiber which helps move waste products through the intestines rapidly, so that they won't turn into cancer-causing substances and stay in contact with the lining of the intestine for long periods of time.

Cereals and whole grain products also contain the mineral selenium which may help to prevent cancer. Population studies have shown that areas of the country where selenium is high in food or in the water have low rates of cancer. Selenium is part of an enzyme in the body which may help combat or prevent cancer.

### Cancer Prevention Tip #14

Avoid cigarettes and other forms of tobacco. Tobacco tar is a potent, cancer-causing substance. When it's applied to the skins of experimental animals, it causes irritation which leads to higher rates of skin cancer in susceptible animals.

Cigarette smoke is the biggest environmental cause of cancer. People who smoke cigarettes or who live or work with people who smoke have higher rates of lung cancer and other cancers than other people. There are over 100,000 deaths from lung cancer in the United States each year. Most of these would never occur in the absence of breathing cigarette smoke.

The rate of lung cancer for ex-smokers goes down dramatically in the years following the time when they stop smoking.

*Cancer Prevention Tip #15*

Avoid alcohol. People who consume high quantities of alcohol have higher rates of cancer than other people. Alcohol may play a direct role in contributing to the development of such cancers as liver cancer. Also, it may take the place of other foods which contain vitamins and other substances which help the body fight and prevent cancer. In other words, alcohol may cause nutritional deficiencies from a lack of other foods that contribute to cancer development.

## Cancer Prevention Tip #16

Avoid artificial sweeteners. Artificial sweeteners containing saccharin have been shown to cause bladder cancer in animals. At present, a number of studies indicate that these same products are fairly safe in humans. Nevertheless, a few studies indicate that bladder cancer in humans, and particularly in human males, may be increased by consuming large amounts of artificial sweeteners containing saccharin.

There is at present no evidence that artificial sweeteners containing aspartame cause cancer in animals or in humans.

## Cancer Prevention Tip #17

Put dietary fiber in your diet. Dietary fiber in the form of bran, whole grain products such as cereal and whole wheat bread, fresh fruits and vegetables can reduce the chances of getting certain kinds of cancer. This has been shown to be true for not just cancer of the colon, but many other kinds of cancer as well. Diets which contain high amounts of foods containing dietary fiber are generally good for overall health as well as for preventing cancer.

Choose foods containing large amounts of vitamin C. Many fruits and vegetables contain large amounts of vitamin C, especially citrus fruits and vegetables like green peppers, cantaloupes, collard greens, broccoli, brussel sprouts, kale, turnip greens, mustard greens, cauliflower, and honeydew melons.

Studies have shown that people who get little vitamin C as food in the diet are prone to develop certain cancers such as cancer of the esophagus or cancer of the larynx.

Massive doses of vitamin C have been promoted as a cancer cure, but research studies about this use are not promising. At best, massive doses of vitamin C may slow down and delay the time of death in terminally ill cancer patients, but this is far from being a cure. However, moderate doses of vitamin C consumed in the form of healthy foods may act as a preventive, since vitamin C helps to activate the immune system which is involved in the body's defenses against cancer.

## Cataracts

Cataracts occur when the lens of the eye becomes cloudy, often with advancing age. It may start when an enzyme system, which helps keep the lens of the eye clear, performs less efficiently with age. Factors contributing to the development of cataracts are:

1. Exposure to ultraviolet light. Wearing sunglasses in bright sunlight or avoiding bright sunlight may be helpful in preventing cataracts.

2. Riboflavin (vitamin B2) deficiency may be one cause of cataracts. There are reports of cataracts diminishing after supplements of riboflavin were taken, but these claims are unconfirmed at this time. On the other hand, taking large doses of the vitamin niacin (vitamin B3) may increase the chances of getting cataracts.

A recent study has shown that people who regularly take acetaminophen or aspirin have 1/2 the rate of cataracts as people who don't take them.

## Chills

Chills are often a symptom of serious disease, infection or a sign of poor circulation. Chills can be caused by vitamin D overdose, which can occur after taking a large amount of a vitamin D supplement or after excessive exposure to sunlight. Sunburn causes the skin to redden and lose heat, and it also makes the skin produce large amounts of vitamin D.

## Choking

There are two good emergency techniques to save a victim who is choking on food. The easiest method is the "tongue pull". First, ask the person to nod his head if he is choking. If he is choking, ask him to stick out his tongue. Grab the tongue with a handkerchief or a napkin or any piece of cloth you can use to get a good grip on it. Then, start to pull the tongue. Then pull it harder and firmer. When pulling on the tongue starts to hurt the victim, the larynx will be pulled upwards, perhaps an inch or so, and the piece of food should become dislodged.

The "tongue pull" isn't as widely known as the "Heimlich Maneuver". In the "Heimlich Maneuver", the rescuer wraps his arms around the victim from behind, clasping his hands. Then the rescuer places the thumbs of the fist of the clasped hands directly under the victim's breastbone and pulls upward with a sharp motion into the area of the victim's diaphragm immediately under his rib cage.

The "Heimlich Maneuver" can be quite successful, but it requires a good deal of skill and strength and may not work on fat people. For this reason, the little known "tongue pull" may be a good initial lifesaving technique. If one technique doesn't work, the other can be tried quickly. It's good to call for emergency medical help at the first sign of trouble even while someone is trying to save a choking victim. Anyone who has been rescued from choking should immediately be taken to a hospital to make sure they are okay and to make sure no food or other foreign object is lodged in the bronchial tubes.

## Circulation Problems

Vitamin E has an anticoagulant effect that may help prevent certain circulation problems. It has been used to treat people with intermittent claudication, poor circulation in the legs, who have a tendency to have leg cramps and form blood clots in the legs.

Niacin is a vasodilator (blood-vessel enlarger). It may improve circulation in the elderly and help keep arms and legs from falling asleep. The effectiveness of this use is unknown, and it may vary.

In diabetics, chromium supplements may aid in treating poor circulation.

Any vitamin or mineral supplements beyond the recommended daily dietary allowance(RDA) should only be taken with a physician's approval.

## Common Cold

The common cold is caused by any number of different viruses affecting the nasal passages and throat. Because of the number of viruses involved, it may be difficult to ever develop a successful cold vaccine. Scientists have tried to overcome this problem by developing interferon sprays which can be manufactured through genetic engineering. Certain of these interferon nasal sprays have the potential of reducing or eliminating colds caused by rhinoviruses and may be available for purchase soon.

The following suggestions have proven successful in combatting or reducing colds and sinus infections.

1. Avoid having children's tonsils removed unless there is severe infection. Tonsils do have a purpose in preventing and combating viral illnesses like colds, so they should not be removed unless necessary. One study has shown that people who have had tonsilectomies have three times as many colds as people who keep their tonsils.

2. Don't become sedentary in the winter.

Regular exercise in the winter may be helpful in keeping your body's thermostat (metabolism) set at a higher level so that your body temperature may be an aide in preventing colds. One theory is that there are far more colds in the winter because the body naturally goes into a sort of semi-hibernation type of metabolism in the winter; because of inactivity in cold weather, the body's thermostat may become set at a lower level. Theoretically, regular exercise can prevent this and help the body maintain the same metabolism it has in the summer when colds are not as prevalent.

3. Avoid exposure to germs from people who have colds. Avoiding exposure doesn't mean getting up and leaving the room everytime someone coughs or sneezes. It does mean washing your hands before meals, or after shaking hands with people who have colds, or changing pillow cases frequently, or using separate towels and washcloths. Recent studies have shown that most colds are transmitted from nose or mouth by hand contact. Interrupting this chain can reduce the chance of catching a cold.

4. Use a humidifier in the cold, dry months of the year. Colds are more prevalent in dry climates. Tissues in the nose dehydrate (dry out) in cold weather, and viruses can escape the

body's defenses better when the surface of tissues in the nose has dried out. Keeping the humidity inside a house at higher levels can be helpful in preventing colds, as well as reducing discomfort from cold symptoms once they appear.

5. Avoid decongestants and antihistamines. Decongestants and antihistamines help reduce cold symptoms, but they may interfere with the body's own defenses. A slightly elevated temperature and a runny nose are the body's way of fighting the cold. When you interfere with these natural defenses, other more serious complications, such as bacterial infections of the sinuses or throat, can develop.

Antihistamines and decongestants may be appropriate for very young children, who are susceptible to ear infections after colds. Cold medications may help the body keep the eustachian tubes to the ear open and prevent ear infections.

6. Wash your hands after blowing your nose or use tissues impregnated with antiviral agents (a relatively new product). You can avoid spreading cold germs to other members of your household by washing your hands frequently, especially after blowing your nose and by discarding tissues properly so that other people will not come in contact with them.

One recent experimental product is a type of tissue for nose blowing and wiping, which is unnoticeably saturated with iodine or other antiviral agents. If tests prove these tissues to be as good as many researchers think they will be, they may play an important role in reducing the spread of colds.

## Confusion

Mental confusion may be caused by advancing age, serious illness, or by a prolonged deficiency of thiamine (vitamin B1), vitamin B12, folic acid or magnesium. Mental confusion may also be a side effect of taking certain prescription drugs.

## Constipation

Constipation is most often caused by a lack of fiber in the diet. High-fiber diets were normal until modern times. Our digestive systems are designed to handle a diet which contains bran, the outer fiber coat of cereal grains. Modern food processing methods remove much fiber from our food, and this leads to constipation. Fiber, or roughage, absorbs a good deal more than its own weight in water; so this "roughage" really becomes "smoothage" in the intestines.

You may think that you aren't constipated if you have a bowel movement every day or so, but you really are if you consume a low-fiber diet. People who eat enough high-fiber food typically pass (without straining) soft, light brown stools, which have little odor. Their movements are regular, about once a day or more. Their breath is sweet since there isn't much absorption of noxious gas through the intestines to the bloodstream, which is then ventilated through the lungs, in constipated people.

Whole grains, fresh fruit, fresh vegetables and unprocessed foods are the best sources of fiber. Some of the foods that naturally provide necessary fiber are: whole grain products, corn, apples, prunes, strawberries, citrus fruit, bananas, figs, pineapples, broccoli, squash, green beans, lettuce, legumes, onions, celery, sweet potatoes, pumpkin, carrots, mushrooms, wheat germ, dates, pecans, sesame seeds, coconuts, sunflower seeds and nuts.

Many prescription and non-prescription drugs can cause constipation as a side effect. Codeine, diuretics (blood pressure reducers), tranquilizers, some antacids, and drugs made of iron preparations like ferrous sulfate are constipating.

Frequent use of laxatives can cause constipation, because laxatives make the body's natural bowel mechanisms insensitive. Using epsom salts or stimulant laxatives may cause people to become dependent on the laxative.

Mineral oil is a laxative commonly used to promote bowel movements by coating the stool and bowel with a film. Prolonged use of mineral oil can lead to a deficiency of certain vitamins like vitamin A, vitamin E or vitamin K. Mineral oil doesn't allow the body to properly absorb these vitamins from food.

Constipation may also be caused by a deficiency of thiamine (Vitamin B1), pantothenic acid (Vitamin B5), Vitamin D, inositol, iron, potassium or calcium.

Vitamin C supplements may have a natural laxative effect.

## Coronary Heart Disease

Many researchers recommend the following natural methods for treating or reducing the chances of developing coronary heart disease (or coronary artery disease).

*Reduce the amount of fat in the diet,* especially saturated fats, which are usually found in meat and dairy products, to 30% of total calorie intake, the level recommended by the American Heart Association; others have recommended even lower levels of from only 10-15%. These levels are substantially lower than the levels found in typical American diets. In a simplified form, they mean eating less meat, dairy products, eggs and other sources of saturated fats and cholesterol, while relying more on starches and low-fat sources of protein such as broiled fish and poultry.

Diets high in protein, as from meat, and low in lysine, as from low fat dairy products, can contribute to heart disease.

*Lower Blood Cholesterol* - High levels of cholesterol in the blood are a risk factor for coronary heart disease. It's a good precaution to measure cholesterol and its HDL (high-density lipoprotein) and LDL (low-density lipoprotein) fractions every time blood is drawn for a physical exam. High LDL levels are harmful, but high HDL levels can help prevent coronary heart disease.

*Gradually Lose Weight* - People who are overweight need to gradually lose weight until normal weight levels are reached and maintained. The fatter an obese person is, the more likely he is to have a heart attack. Excess pounds put extra strain on the heart.

*Do Not Smoke* - Quit smoking to reduce chances of heart disease. Heavy cigarette smokers have twice the death rate from coronary heart disease as non-smokers. Non-smokers who live in the same house with a heavy cigarette smoker have higher death rates from coronary heart disease than non-smokers who do not live with a person who smokes. Heavy cigarette smokers have a life expectancy as much as 10 years less than that of non-smokers.

*Get Moderate Physical Exercise* - Brisk walking is the type of exercise recommended by most doctors. It's preferred because it puts a moderate amount of stress on the heart and lungs and serves to strengthen them, while not exerting them to the point where it's likely that a heart attack would occur.

A recent study shows that older people with painful foot problems, which prevented normal standing or walking activities, had extremely high rates of heart attacks, several times higher than expected.

It's a paradox that while many studies show that regular, sustained "aerobic" exercise strengthens the heart, helps the circulation, and is a positive benefit, they also indicate that sudden, unaccustomed bursts of exercise can lead to heart attacks in susceptible people.

*Avoid Stressful Situations* - Avoid pressure in the office, arguments, and heavy strenuous exercise like shoveling snow.

*Lower High Blood Pressure* - Reducing high blood pressure helps lessen the chance of developing coronary artery disease.

See: **Blood Pressure, High.**

*Doctor Prescribed Daily Aspirin* - One aspirin tablet per day can cut heart attacks by 20% for some people who have already had a heart attack, and as much as 50% in men who have unstable angina, according to the FDA (U.S. Food and Drug Administration). People already undergoing treatment for a past heart attack or unstable angina should consult with their doctor before starting daily aspirin therapy.

Aspirin inhibits the action of small cell fragments in the blood called platelets, which have a role in blood clotting. In this way, aspirin is thought to decrease the likelihood of having a heart attack. A heart attack usually results when a clot blocks the blood flow to the heart muscle.

It remains to be seen if aspirin will help people who have not had heart attacks but who may be developing coronary heart disease.

*Avoid Alcohol* - Alcoholism or heavy consumption of alcoholic beverages is a definite risk factor which leads to increased rates of heart attacks.

*Eat Salt Water Fish* - The oil found in some fresh water fish and all salt water fish has recently been discovered to be beneficial in raising HDL levels in the blood. Recent population studies show that people who eat substantial amounts of cold water fish like trout, salmon, mackerel or cod have lower rates of coronary heart disease than other people, even if the total amount of fat in the diet remains about the same. These new studies suggest that the addition of fish to the diet, and especially the replacement of much red meat and dairy products with fish, could reduce the chance of developing coronary heart disease.

*Pay Attention To Heredity* - People who come from families where their parents or other close relatives have had coronary heart disease are at greater risk than people who come from families with low rates of coronary heart disease. Although heredity is not controllable, the presence of coronary heart disease in close family members is a risk factor which indicates that it is more likely to develop; all possible precautions should be taken.

*Vitamins and Minerals* - Pyridoxine (vitamin B6) deficiency may contribute to coronary heart disease. Pyridoxine supplementation may be especially helpful in preventing heart and artery disease for people who eat high-protein diets. When meat is cooked, it loses much of its pyridoxine which could have been used by the body to help break down by-products of methionine, one of the amino acids found in protein. By-products of methionine are thought to damage the arteries and cause heart disease much like the process which is involved to a much greater extent in homocystinuria (a hereditary enzyme-deficiency disease). Taking small supplements of pyridoxine with each meal containing cooked meat may help to prevent some coronary heart disease.

Studies by Kurt A. Oster, M.D. and others indicate that folic acid may be helpful in the treatment and prevention of heart disease. Larger, controlled studies are necessary to confirm these studies.

Another medical doctor states that folic acid may stop the progress of coronary heart disease not only by neutralizing xanthine oxidase,but also by restoring a substance which repairs damage to arteries and helps stop the fatty buildup which is found in hardening of the arteries.

Magnesium or selenium deficiency may result in coronary heart disease.

*For Women Only* - A National Institute of Health study concluded that women should take estrogen during mid-life and especially during menopause to lower risk of heart disease. The death rate from heart disease in estrogen users was 1/3 the rate of women who did not take estrogen. However, reports published in the New England Journal of Medicine challenge this conclusion.

Self-treatment, especially in the case of a serious illness like coronary artery disease, is not a good idea. Even though natural methods of preventing coronary artery disease may be helpful there is no substitute for management defying skilled physician if you already have coronary artery disease or if you ever had a heart attack.

Please consult your physician before changing any established treatment program for coronary heart disease.

**Cystitis:** See Bladder Infections

**Dental Problems**

Rates of tooth decay in the western world are higher now than some centuries ago. Dental decay and disease have greatly increased in other countries within a decade or two of adopting the eating habits of western civilization. A brief look at the historical emergence of dental disease with respect to diet might give some insight into dental health.

In studies of tooth decay among British

people living from 3000 B.C. to A.D. 800, teeth having cavities were rarely, if ever, discovered. During these periods in Britain, the following incidence of dental cavities is reported:

| | |
|---|---|
| Neolithic | 4% |
| Roman (1st century A.D.) | 12% |
| Saxon | 5% |

The rise in tooth decay during the Roman period is probably due, according to one historian, to the fact that fine-ground flour and sweets were widely available for consumption during that period. The incidence fell again during the Anglo-Saxon period but rose again in the 16th century, as did the consumption of refined carbohydrate foods, and has been rising ever since. The historical pattern of emergence of dental cavities in America is similar to that in Britain.

Very low incidences of dental disease have been reported among people living in a primitive culture and consuming a diet of unrefined foodstuffs. Studies have shown that in rural Alaska, China, Egypt, Greenland, India, Kenya, Kuria Muria islands of the Middle East, Mexico, Peru, Morocco, North America, Sudan, Tristan da Cunha and Uganda, the average rate of decayed, missing or filled teeth was less than 2 per person compared with 10-11 per person in the urban United States.

There is much evidence to suggest that

eating a diet consisting largely of refined carbohydrate foods is a major causative factor in tooth decay and dental disease. A 1972 study of American school children showed that those who were free of cavities did not eat sugar-containing foods or else ate them infrequently. A 1951 survey in China turned up an extremely low incidence of dental cavities among 3,349 persons aged 12-27 years. Their regular diet contained no sugar.

Two studies from opposite poles of the earth seem to point to the fact that heredity, race or geography have little, if any, effect on tooth decay. In 1972, two men studied a group of Eskimos living in northern Alaska whose regular diet was fish, marine mammals, and birds. In 1953, a small trading post had been opened by a white trader. Three more stores were opened from 1957-65, and sugar and other refined foods became a regular part of their diet. In 1955-57, 75% of the people had cavity-free permanent teeth, but by 1965 not a single person was free of dental cavities. The average rate of decayed, missing or filled teeth had increased four times in those 8-10 years.

A study dating from 1932 of the islanders of Tristan da Cunha near the South Pole presents a very convincing case for the role of refined foods in causing tooth decay. In 1932 their diet consisted mainly of fish, potatoes, milk, eggs and green vegetables. Eighty-three percent of the population was free from cavities or any missing teeth: children aged 1-5 years had no dental cavities; no one under the age of 21 had cavities in permanent teeth. Between the years 1932 and 1937, ships came to the island with increased frequency, bringing with them goods containing sugar and refined flour. The rate of islanders with no cavities or missing teeth dropped in those years to only 50%. By 1952, with a fishing station and store well- established, only 22% of the population had no cavities or no missing teeth; 32% of children aged 1-5 years had dental cavities. Sugar and flour had become essential foodstuffs, and the average yearly consumption of sugar per family was over 105 kilograms.(Yearly intake of sugar in the average U.S. family today is over 150 kilograms.)

Similar trends toward increased dental disease with increased consumption of refined carbohydrate foods have been observed among other groups of people, such as Africans, Navajo Indians in the United States, and South Arabians.

Just as refined carbohydrate foods have been shown to increase incidences of dental decay, so unrefined carbohydrate foods have been shown to actually offer protection against the solubility of the tooth enamel and against dental cavities.

Sugar cane juice, oatmeal, wheat bran, wheat germ, and hulls of oats, peanuts and pecans are associated with factors which reduce the solubility of tooth enamel. Just how these factors operate in a protective manner is not clear; one explanation is that it takes longer to chew unrefined foods and so they stay in contact with the teeth for a longer period of time. Also, the longer chewing period promotes increased saliva flow, which has a flushing effect on the teeth and, in the presence of unrefined foods, has a high buffering power.

### Non-Dietary Ways To Prevent Or Clear Up Dental Problems Before It Is Too Late

1. Avoid mouthwash. Most commercial mouthwashes can cause sore gums and tongues. Many people who use mouthwashes develop mouth ulcers or other forms of mouth or tongue irritation. Use of mouthwashes may also be related to the development of cancer. One study of eleven victims of head and neck cancer who were neither smokers or drinkers disclosed that ten of them had used mouthwash at least twice daily for more than twenty years. Although it's not proven, mouthwashes may contain substances that can cause cancer in certain susceptible individuals.

People can gain the benefits of using mouthwashes and stop the risk simply by using their toothbrush on the tongue and mouth as well as the teeth and gum line. This helps to remove bacteria which can cause odor and leave a bad taste in the mouth.

2. Prevent gum disease by changing from toothpaste to a salt solution. Dr. Paul Keyes who has done work at the National Institute of Dental Research states that he has never seen a case of gum disease in a person  who has regularly used salt or a soda dentifrice. He advocates brushing with a solution made by putting water in a glass and pouring enough salt in it so that no more will dissolve after stirring. Other dentists recommend brushing with baking soda; it also has a scouring effect that helps clean the gum line where gum disease and decay start around plaque that forms there.  Dr. Keyes states that his program  is also good for treating early stages of pyorrhea.

Incidentally, severe cases of gum disease are often treated successfully without expensive surgery by dentists using scaling tools and  a diluted hydrogen peroxide solution or an antibiotic.  Use of diluted 1% hydrogen peroxide may be effective, but it is not generally recommended for home use in treating or preventing gum disease. Many dentists achieve rates of success which are at least equal to,or better than, gum surgery by using Dr. Keye's techniques.

Vitamin C deficiency can increase, or lead to, bleeding or swelling of the gums or aggravate gum disease. Many smokers lose their teeth because smoking seems to deplete vitamin C levels in the body, especially in the mouth. This leads to susceptibility to gum disease, tooth loss, and decay.

## How To Get Rid Of A Toothache

Any toothache is a sign of a serious dental problem which should be treated by a dentist. In the meantime, a drop of clove oil applied to the cavity with a piece of cotton on a toothpick is remarkably effective in eliminating the pain. Once the pain is gone, don't assume that clove oil will fix the problem. Pain is a symptom of a serious dental problem which should be treated immediately.

## Depression

Mental depression can have many symptoms such as fatigue, "laziness", an inability to start or finish work, feelings of sadness, hopelessness or irritability. These symptoms are normal for everyone at times, and most people get better within a few days or weeks.

Endogenous mental depression is prolonged, and it may not be clearly caused by grief or mental shocks. Prescription drug side effects frequently cause depression. Blood pressure reducers, sleeping pills, tranquilizers and many other drugs may cause depression. Overdoses of certain vitamins, especially niacinamide, can cause depression. Allergies to foods, like corn or gluten, can cause depression, especially if the allergy causes intestinal problems which interfere with the absorption of vitamins. Eating foods containing large amounts of sugar or flour may cause low blood sugar levels and depression. Vitamin deficiencies, especially deficiencies of B vitamins, can cause depression. Alcohol causes mental depression. Withdrawal from drugs, including caffeine, nicotine and alcohol, may cause depression.

Because depression can be a symptom of serious disease and because depressed people may commit suicide, it's appropriate to seek help from a qualified medical doctor. Doctors may treat severe depression with antidepressants or psychotherapy. Studies show that a combination of antidepressants, psychotherapy and loving care by friends and relatives is often helpful.

Bright indoor lighting helps some people fight depression in the winter by stimulating the brain and the pineal gland. Vigorous exercise for a few minutes a day stimulates the brain and helps combat depression.

**Diarrhea**

Diarrhea can be caused by excessive amounts of vitamins, certain prescription drugs, or more commonly by an infection which may be mild or serious. Diarrhea can also be a symptom of serious intestinal disease. Anyone with diarrhea should consult a physician to make sure that nothing serious is wrong. Persistent diarrhea from an infection or parasite may be treated with drugs. If nothing serious is wrong, several steps may help to minimize or eliminate diarrhea.

1.

Avoid taking vitamins or minerals on an empty stomach and check carefully to see if diarrhea is related to any prescription drug you're taking. If it is a side effect of a drug, consult your physician about changing your medication.

Diarrhea may also be caused by certain foods, such as dietetic products containing sorbitol or mannitol. Milk products also cause problems for certain individuals who have difficulty digesting lactose. If lactose intolerance is a problem, you should avoid milk products containing lactose or use a predigested type of milk to which the enzyme lactase has been added. Over-the-counter liquids containing bismuth may be helpful for common diarrhea.

Diarrhea may cause dehydration. Serious fluid loss, especially in children, may have to be treated in a hospital with intravenous therapy. Moderate fluid loss can be treated under a physcian's guidance at home by taking plenty of liquids plus potassium chloride, which is found in some brands of "light" salt, and sodium bicarbonate in moderate amounts.

**Diverticular Disease**

Diverticular disease is the out-ballooning of areas of the intestine into little pockets, in which fecal matter can lodge and cause infection. Many doctors who treat people with diverticular disease now recommend that they eat a diet which is high in dietary fiber or take a fiber supplement. The types of fiber recommended are the mushy types such as psyllium seed products or oat bran, as well as whole grain products. Hard types of fiber such as popcorn should be avoided.

People with diverticulosis or diverticulitis experience far fewer relapses if they consume appropriate dietary fiber daily, than if they eat a diet like the traditional American diet which is quite low in dietary fiber. Although the problems caused by diverticular disease will not disappear on a high fiber diet or after taking a fiber supplement daily, in most cases, they can be minimized and controlled so that surgery or antibiotic treatment can be avoided.

## Ear Noises

Tinnitus or ringing in the ears is a serious problem for millions of Americans. In most cases, the cause is unknown and incurable, but some cases can be helped significantly by the following health tips.

1. Avoid alcohol, nicotine, marijuana, or caffeine.

2. Avoid loud noises such as jack hammers, construction machinery, noise from industrial machinery, airplane motors, unmuffled racing car motors, lawn mowers and loud amplified music from loudspeakers.

3. Certain prescription drugs, including tranquilizers, oral contraceptives, quinine and

aspirin products, can cause ringing in the ears.

4. Ringing in the ears is a frequent side effect of vitamin D overdose, which can occur after overexposure to sunlight, which produces sunburn, as well as after taking large doses of vitamin D supplements.

5. Zinc supplements have been reported to help some cases of hearing loss and ringing in the ears.

### Fatigue

Fatigue may be a symptom of a serious disease which needs medical treatment. A physician should be consulted if fatigue continues.

Fatigue may be caused by a deficiency of certain vitamins or minerals, including thiamine (vitamin B1), riboflavin (vitamin B2), niacin (vitamin B3), pantothenic acid (vitamin B5, vitamin B12, vitamin C or folic acid.

Over-consumption of caffeine may cause fatigue when the effects of the drug wear off, especially early in the morning. Monitor the number of caffeine-containing drinks (colas, coffee, tea) that you have daily, and start eliminating them.

Taking vitamin E in doses larger than the recommended daily dietary allowance (RDA) is reported to sometimes cause fatigue.

Fatigue, especially in women, is often related to low levels of iron, particularly in women who have heavy menstrual flow. Eating foods rich in iron, such as raisins, may be helpful. Iron supplements, particularly in large doses, can sometimes be dangerous, so natural sources of iron are preferred. Consult your physician.

Taking extra vitamin C or the mineral manganese has been reported to reduce fatigue in some people.

### Feeling, Loss of

Feeling loss or numbness may be a symptom of a serious disease which needs medical treatment.

Loss of feeling combined with tingling or burning sensations may be a symptom of lack of thiamine (vitamin B1).

A deficiency of vitamin B12 can also lead to numbness and tingling in the feet.

Niacin (vitamin B3) may improve circulation in the elderly thus keeping arms and legs from falling asleep. The overall effectiveness of this use of niacin is unknown, and it may vary from person to person .

## Fertility

There are many causes of infertility, and there are many ways that fertility can be increased so that childless couples can have children.

Infertility in males may be caused by low sperm counts or a reduced ability of sperm to swim. Sperm counts can sometimes be increased by switching from wearing jockey shorts to boxer shorts or by avoiding hot tubs, steam rooms or hot tub baths. Even small increases in temperature in the groin can lower sperm counts and reduce fertility in men.

Past or current infections in men and women can interfere with fertility. One study revealed that as many as one-third of infertile patients seeking help at a hospital were diagnosed as having T-mycoplasma infections. These infections were treated with an antibiotic, doxycycline, which was given to patients and their spouses for four weeks. Most of the infected childless couples were able to successfully conceive following this treatment.

Past infections, particularly from venereal diseases, may create tissue scarring in the reproductive system, resulting in infertility.

Many childless couples are helped by taking fertility drugs. One type of drug is an estrogen look-a-like which fools the body into thinking that it is time to ovulate, so the body puts out extra amounts of follicle-stimulating hormone (FSH). This drug, Clomid®, is effective in treating more than half the cases of infertility which are related to hormonal imbalances in the female partner. As a last resort, some women with hormonal imbalances take the drug Pergonal®, but Pergonal® can cause a high incidence of multiple births which may be dangerous to the mother and the offspring.

## Fever Blisters

Fever blisters are caused by a herpes simplex virus infection. Infection with herpes simplex type I or herpes simplex type II is rather common. Blisters may break out in the mouth or in the genital area, and they tend to recur in many people. Herpes infections can be transmitted sexually or through other methods of contact. Herpes simplex type II is the more common causal organism in venereal (sexually transmitted) herpes.

People with herpes infections may suffer frequent outbreaks of blisters in the mouth or genital area, which can be quite painful or which may be mild in nature. The herpes virus seems to hide in nerve tissue and to break out, causing blisters, when conditions are right for its multiplication.

Recently, researchers have discovered that the amino acid lysine helps prevent herpes outbreaks by keeping the virus contained, while the amino acid arginine actually promotes herpes outbreaks. Studies are now underway which indicate that diets high in lysine and low in arginine can, in many cases, control or prevent herpes outbreaks.

The best dietary source of lysine is skim milk and skim milk products. Nuts are the best source of arginine, so they should be avoided by people who are prone to get fever blisters. Additionally, some people advocate taking lysine supplements. One study has shown that this may be effective for preventing fever blisters. Since lysine is an acid, it should be taken after eating food and drinking adequate amounts of liquid so that it will not irritate the stomach.

**Gallbladder Disease:** see **Gallstones**

**Gallstones**

Gallstones are common in all western countries for which there are available statistics. They affect every social class, and there is an increasing incidence among younger people. Gallstone formation formerly had been regarded as a disease of the middle-aged and elderly. Women are about twice as prone as men to form gallstones.

Gallstones are not common in underdeveloped countries. In fact, there is little published information on the frequency of gallstones in such countries. That fact in itself suggests the rarity of the disease, since absence of a disease will normally evoke less comment than its presence. Available information from various countries (Africa in particular) on gallstone incidence there shows how rare or nonexistent the disease is.

An autopsy survey in Uganda in 1964 showed gallstones present in only 1.35% of subjects aged 35-64.

In Ghana a study of 4935 autopsies reported not a single case of gallstones.

At Ibadan University Hospital over a 5 year period, only 27 patients were admitted because of gallstones, and such patients tended to be obese, wealthy, and consumers of a westernized diet.

Dennis Burkitt, in his 17 years of surgical practice in East Africa, reported operating on only two patients with gallstones, one of whom was a queen and very likely eating a typically western, low-fiber diet.

High-fiber diets are the norm in countries with a low incidence of gallstones. Low-fiber diets are consumed where there is a high incidence of gallstones. Studies done by Pomare and Heaton in 1973 and 1974 suggest that a high-fiber diet may lessen the risk of gallstone formation. The addition of bran to the diet seemed to interfere with the appearance of a secondary bile salt which makes the bile more saturated with cholesterol and keeps cholesterol from being secreted into the intestine. Since almost all gallstones in the people of western countries consist of cholesterol, this research has important implications in the prevention of gallstone formation.

It can be seen from studies of people who have become more westernized that the incidence of gallstones increases with urbanization. This is graphically illustrated in the Canadian Eskimo. Up until about 10 or so years ago, gallstones were rarely seen among these people. However, Eskimos have been rapidly adopting western habits into their lifestyle, and in at least one town where western culture predominates, operations for gallbladder disease have outnumbered all other operative procedures undertaken in the past ten years.

Because of increasing evidence, eating

whole grain foods and bran and avoiding high-fat diets should be helpful in the prevention of gallstone formation.

If you already have gallstones, you may be able to avoid a gallbladder operation through one of the experimental methods now being investigated. One new method of crushing gallstones without having to endure an operation is to use a giant ultrasonic machine called a lithotripser, which uses "sound waves" to break up and crush kidney stones in the body. Although the use of the lithotripser for crushing gallstones is new and experimental, this use may become more widespread in the future. Many major medical centers now have lithotripsers.

Other promising techniques of avoiding gallbladder operations involve administering certain substances which may dissolve the gallstones.

### Glaucoma

Glaucoma is caused by a hereditary tendency which leads to a build-up of fluids and pressure within the eye, which may ultimately lead to blindness. Glaucoma is treated medically with drugs and surgery.

Glaucoma may be aggravated by taking large doses of vitamin D in the form of supplements or by heavy exposure to sunlight. Large doses of niacin may also aggravate glaucoma. Supplements of vitamin A or choline, as well as vitamin C supplements, have been used to help in the treatment of glaucoma, but the effectiveness of such use is questionable.

### Hair, Gray

In 1980, Dr. Abram Hoffer, a medical doctor who advocates large doses of vitamins in the treatment of certain disorders, claimed that vitamin E supplementation returned his gray hair back to its normal color. Another researcher has reported that taking very high doses of para-aminobenzoic acid darkened his gray hair. Other researchers claim that zinc, pantothenic acid, and folic acid may prevent graying of the hair or restore hair color to gray hair.

The overall effectiveness of vitamin supplements for preventing gray hair or restoring color to hair that is already gray is unknown and unproven. Taking vitamins at the recommended daily dietary allowance levels is okay, but large doses of vitamins should be taken cautiously and with a physician's consent, because of the possibility of serious side effects.

**Hair Loss**

Most hair loss is caused by an hereditary gene which is expressed fully in males but not fully in females. Although both males and females lose hair, full hereditary baldness usually occurs only in males who have a double dose of the gene from both parents.

Uncommon loss of hair may be caused by deficiency of riboflavin (vitamin B2), biotin or copper, or else by overdoses of vitamin A or selenium. Taking inositol, biotin, or zinc supplements or using ointments containing these substances is sometimes advocated for reducing hair loss or restoring hair that is already lost, but the effectiveness of such treatments is disappointing. Estrogen cremes have been used to reduce hair loss, but they may cause breast enlargement or other side effects.

**Hardening of the Arteries:** see
**Coronary Heart Disease**

**Headaches**

Headaches may have many causes. Mild headaches that are not symptoms of a serious disease are usually treated with aspirin or acetaminophen. Long lasting, frequent or severe headaches or headaches associated with other problems may be symptoms of a serious disease, so they're a signal to see your doctor. If headaches are not a symptom of another serious disease, they can be treated naturally in a number of different ways depending on what kind of headaches they are.

Migraine headaches are severe headaches which can be associated with other symptoms, such as nausea or visual disturbances such as seeing flashes of light. Migraine pain usually is localized on one side of the head. Migraines can often be avoided by avoiding the "trigger" for the headache. Exposure to sunshine seems to cause about 30% of all migraines. An allergic reaction to various foods, especially milk products, may cause many other cases of migraine. The elimination of suspected foods from the diet can bring dramatic relief to many sufferers. Other migraines are caused by increases in estrogen levels near the end of monthly menstrual cycles or after taking birth control pills.

The most promising new natural treatment for migraines is to take magnesium supplements. Magnesium is usually deficient in the American diet, and magnesium supplements like magnesium chloride or dolomite, which is composed of calcium carbonate and magnesium carbonate, are quite helpful to many migaine sufferers, especially women who suffer from migraines during pregnancy or near the end of their monthly cycles.

Physicians usually treat migraines with antihistamines, decongestants or caffeine and ergot-based drugs which constrict the enlarged blood vessels in the skull that cause migraines. If caffeine and ergot-based preparations don't work, physicians often prescribe beta-blockers o calcium channel blockers, drugs which are generally used as blood pressure reducers Prescription drugs can cause severe side effects. Natural methods for treating migraines are preferred if they will work.

Headaches can be caused by pressure to the neck or head. Wearing swimming goggles, wearing tight fitting glasses or tight fitting collars bring on headaches in many people.

Headaches may occur as side effects of taking or withdrawing from various drugs or vitamins. Birth control pills are especially apt to cause headaches in some people, and caffeine withdrawal, such as not getting a morning cup of coffee by someone who regularly drinks coffee, often will cause a headache. Deficiencies of certain vitamins or overdoses of certain vitamins also can cause headaches.

Smoking and drinking alcohol frequently

causes headaches. Withdrawal from frequent smoking and drinking usually causes headaches but only for one or two weeks.

Headaches may occur as a result of a sinus infection or sinus blockage from allergies. Antibiotics, decongestants or surgery are often prescribed by doctors to treat sinus headaches. Simple over-the-counter sinus decongestants often work well to relieve sinus headaches.

Tension headaches are probably the most common kind of headache. They can often be treated successfully by relaxing muscles in the neck. Neck and shoulder massage by another person or stretching neck muscles by bending the head forward at an angle alternately to the right and to the left while gently pulling down on the back of the head to stretch neck muscles may help. Also, moderate exercise can often relieve tension headache pain.

### Hearing Loss

Hearing loss can be caused by many conditions, including changes associated with aging, heart conditions, viral infections, bacterial infections, stroke, exposure to loud noises, tumors, some drugs, excessive ear wax, head injuries or physical changes within the middle or inner ears.

If hearing loss is caused by bacterial infection, treatment with antibiotics may clear up the infection and help restore hearing. Many children who have persistent fluid levels behind the eardrum and ear infections can have their hearing restored by having tubes implanted through the eardrums to drain the fluid. This condition, known as otitis media, is related to chronic ear infections. Elimination of sugar in drinks or baby bottles in young children can also clear up recurrent ear infections by denying harmful microrganisms the sugar which promotes their growth.

In adults, particularly older adults, hearing loss may be the result of nerve damage. Zinc supplements have been shown, in many cases, to reverse a certain type of progressive inner ear nerve loss where people are deficient in zinc or in some cases where people also suffer from ringing in the ears. In a recent study, 50 hearing loss patients with a confirmed zinc deficiency were given large doses of zinc, ten times the recommended daily dietary allowance. All of the patients in this study experienced improvement in their hearing, and the ones who suffered from ringing in the ears also experienced improvement. Large doses of zinc like those used in this study should only be given upon a physician's advice because of the possibility of serious side effects.

Many people with progressive hearing loss can be helped by eliminating substances from the diet which cause allergic deafness. If deafness is caused by a food allergy, improvement can be dramatic and total. Doctors start this treatment by first giving an anti-allergy drug to the patient. If allergic reactions are causing the problem, the patient may regain his hearing within an hour of receiving the anti-allergy drug. Later, once the offending food substance is identified and avoided, the restoration of hearing may be permanent.

People with hearing loss caused by a deterioration of the bone in the inner ear called otospongeosis have been helped by fluoride supplements. Fluoride supplements of up to 10 times the recommended daily allowance have restored hearing over a period of time to some extent in these patients. Caution: large doses of fluoride can be extremely poisonous, and any fluoride supplementation beyond the recommended daily allowance can have serious side effects and should only be undertaken with close monitoring by a physician.

Finally, some cases of hearing loss can be corrected by doing things as simple as having a physician remove excessive ear wax, avoiding loud noises from machinery or loudspeakers, or trying an alternate prescription drug if hearing loss is the side effect of medication that someone is taking.

## Heartburn

Heartburn occurs when acid from the stomach forces its way up into the lower part of the esophagus. The esophagus has a circular sphincter muscle which closes to keep acid in the stomach, but it may become detached or lose some of its strength, allowing stomach acid to escape. If a medical checkup doesn't disclose serious disease, heartburn can usually be treated successfully by natural means.

One of the chief causes of heartburn is smoking cigarettes or using other tobacco products such as snuff, smokeless tobacco, pipes or cigars. Nicotine in tobacco products weakens the sphincter muscle.

After smoking, the next most common cause is a low-fiber diet. Diets which are low in fiber promote constipation which can push up on the stomach and cause heartburn. Adding bran and whole grain products to the diet can help relieve heartburn for many people.

Coffee consumption increases stomach acid secretions, so it may play a role in causing heartburn.

Eating certain foods, such as fried foods and other things which are irritating to the stomach, can cause heartburn.

Eating before bedtime or eating large meals can cause heartburn. Being overweight increases abdominal pressure and can contribute to heartburn. Pregnancy causes heartburn in many mothers-to-be toward the later part of their pregnancy. Tight belts or girdles can increase pressure on the stomach and cause heartburn.

Eliminating causes of heartburn as listed above can have a dramatic effect on relieving most cases of heartburn. Most physicians recommend antacid preparations for combating heartburn. Of course, antacid preparations can help, but they are less desirable than taking natural steps to eliminate the causes of heartburn. The types of antacids which coat the stomach and which are dispensed in liquid form are most effective in relieving heartburn.

See also: **Hiatus Hernia**

**Heart Disease:** see **Coronary Heart Disease**

**Heatstroke**

Heatstroke usually occurs because of

overexposure to the sun or because of exercising vigorously in hot temperatures and high humidity. Heat stroke is more severe than heat exhaustion. In heat exhaustion, the body will usually recover on its own; but in heatstroke, the body sometimes goes into very high temperature, followed by shock and death of body tissues which may prove fatal. Emergency medical aid is essential in treating heatstroke.

Heatstroke is more apt to occur in young children than in adults and in people who become dehydrated after exercising in warm weather.

Certain drugs, combined with high humidity and warm temperatures, may lead to heatstroke. Anticholinergics, like certain asthma medications, and antipsychotic drugs, such as phenothiazines, affect the central nervous system and distort the body's natural thermostat.

Extra care to avoid overheating during exercise should be taken by people who use drugs which can cause decreased sweating. These include Belladenal®, Bellergal®, Chardonna-2®, Dicyclomine®, Donnatal®, Donnazyme®. Kinesed®, Librax®, Wigran-PS®, antidyskinetics and drugs to treat Parkinson's Disease.

## Hemorrhoids

Hemorrhoids are enlarged, dilated veins of the rectal and anal passages. They can occur at any age, but they are found more often as people get older.

Most hemorrhoids are caused by eating a diet which is low in dietary fiber, like fiber found in bran and whole grain products, and in many vegetables such as corn and beans.

Not only are hemorrhoids caused by lack of dietary fiber, but their symptoms can be relieved in almost all cases by putting fiber back into the diet.

This little known health secret is simple and effective in treating hemorrhoids. All you have to do is start the day with a good whole grain cereal for breakfast, eat a sandwich on some whole grain bread for lunch and eat lots of fresh vegetables and whole grain rolls for supper. Almost everyone who does this ceases to be bothered by hemorrhoid symptoms within a few days or few weeks.

Unfortunately, the weakness in the veins which causes hemorrhoids will remain even when fiber is added back into the diet. If a person who has suffered from hemorrhoids in the past ceases to be conscientious in following a diet that contains an adequate amount of dietary fiber, the hemorrhoids will flare up once again.

**Herpes:** see **Fever Blisters**

## Hiatus Hernia

Hiatus hernia occurs when the sphincter muscle, which keeps food and acid from the stomach from being regurgitated up into the esophagus, becomes separated from the surrounding tissues so that it doesn't do its job effectively. Then, acid irritates the esophagus and throat and causes "heartburn".

Hiatus hernia can be caused by smoking, constipation, or obesity; and it can often be relieved by giving up smoking, eating a high-fiber diet, or losing weight. Hiatus hernia which occurs because of extra abdominal pressure during pregnancy can often be treated successfully with antacids.

The health tips for relieving heartburn also apply to relieving hiatus hernia. The two conditions are closely related. Heartburn can occur without the muscle damage of hiatus hernia, but hiatus hernia rarely occurs without heartburn.

Hiatus hernia can be caused by serious disease, so see your doctor. Severe cases of hiatus hernia which do not respond to natural methods can be corrected by an operation. Natural methods, which are usually successful, should be tried first, with surgery considered as a final option.

See also: **Heartburn.**

**Hiccups**

Hiccups occur as the result of an involuntary spasm of the diaphragm, the big muscle under the lungs which regulates breathing. Hiccups usually will stop if the concentration of carbon dioxide in the bloodstream reaches a fairly high level. The first health secret for stopping hiccups is simply to hold your breath as long as you possibly can, even through several involuntary hiccups. A second method for increasing carbon dioxide concentration in the blood is to breathe in and out of a paper bag for as long as you can, rebreathing the same air that you have exhaled. A third method is to hold your breath and drink a glass of water with many small sips.

If increasing the concentration of carbon dioxide in the blood is not feasible, as it may not be in small children, try swallowing a teaspoon of dry sugar or swallowing dry crackers. The resulting tickling sensation in the back of the throat may stop the hiccups.

**High Blood Pressure:** see **Blood Pressure, High**

## Hip Fracture

Hip fractures often occur in older people. When an older person breaks his or her hip, death often follows because of complications of being bedridden while recovering from the broken hip. Older folks who are bedridden often get blood clots, which may travel to the lungs or to the brain and cause serious injury or strokes.

A good health secret for older folks is to make sure that hazardous areas are made safer. The first step is to put non-skid strips on the bottom of the bathtub and to make sure that there is a good handrail near it. Next, remove loose throw rugs from the house, especially from hallways where a person may slip while making a turn. Finally, handrails should be put up beside all stairs and steps.

There are also ways to strengthen the actual bone tissue so that a fall in an older person may not cause a fracture. Addition of calcium and vitamin D to the diet, within the recommended daily dietary allowance, often helps older people combat the thinning of the bone. Bone degeneration happens in osteoporosis which occurs, especially in women, as they get older.

See: Osteoporosis.

**Hypertension:** see **Blood Pressure, High**

**Impotence**

Impotence usually occurs for physical reasons and not psychological reasons. It occurs more often as people get older. Impotence is often a side effect of alcohol or prescription drugs, such as medication for high blood pressure. Lowering blood pressure by natural means may enable a doctor to take a patient off the blood pressure medicine which may be causing or contributing to impotence.

Taking vitamin E has been advocated by some people to increase sexual function and to combat impotence. Vitamin E is proven to increase fertility in some people, but there is no evidence that it increases sexual drive or reduces impotence. As a matter of fact, one study showed that taking large doses of vitamin E may cause reduced sexual function.

Taking zinc supplements has been reported to improve some cases of impotence, but its effectiveness is unproven. Large doses of zinc supplements can be dangerous, so any zinc supplementation should be within the recommended daily dietary allowance (15 mg. per day for adults).

Impotence often is a consequence of nerve damage during operations for removal of cancerous prostate glands, because much of the surrounding tissue is also removed. However, impotence rarely occurs as a result of operations to relieve constriction from an enlarged prostate gland which is non-cancerous, since this operation is less radical. Impotence caused by nerve damage from an operation cannot be corrected, except by unusual methods, such as surgical implants in the penis.

Good overall health is the best way to combat many cases of impotence. Regular, daily exercise, keeping weight under control and eating a healthy diet with lots of whole grain products and little fat can improve overall health and perhaps, in some cases, counteract a tendency towards impotence.

A mild stimulant like caffeine in coffee sometimes will help reduce impotence.

### Indigestion

Indigestion, if it is not caused by an infectious illness or other serious disease, is usually caused by intolerance to foods. Milk and milk products, especially those containing lactose, are chief offenders in many cases of indigestion. Other foods such as corn, processed meats, spicy foods, tomatoes, etc. may cause indigestion. See your doctor to make sure indigestion is not caused by serious disease and, if not, start eliminating foods from the diet to see if you can find the culprits.

Nutritional deficiencies may cause indigestion. Diets which are low in pantothenic acid (vitamin B5) or other vitamins can lead to indigestion.

On the other hand, taking large doses of certain vitamins can cause indigestion. Vitamin C in the form of ascorbic acid can irritate the stomach and cause nausea, indigestion and even stomach ulcers. Taking vitamin E in doses larger than the recommended daily dietary allowance can cause indigestion at times. Vitamin supplements should always be taken on a full stomach to avoid irritation of the stomach lining, and vitamin supplements in doses larger than the recommended daily dietary allowance (RDA) should be avoided if they cause indigestion.

Indigestion may be caused by several over-the-counter or prescription drugs, including: aspirin, antihistamines, anti-inflammatory drugs used to treat arthritis, some antibiotics, uric acid inhibitors used to treat gout, sedatives, blood vessel enlarging drugs, narcotics, antidepressants and pain relievers.

**Infertility:** see **Fertility**

**Insect Stings and Bites**

Insect stings can be relieved by first removing the stinger with tweezers and then immediately applying a small dab of bleach with a swab to the top of the sting, but not to much of the surrounding area. A dab of ammonia works well for mosquito bites, flea bites, or gnat bites. A paste made of meat tenderizer and water also works well on bites and stings.

Wasps, bees, and hornets will rarely sting anyone unless they are bothered. You don't have to run from them unless they are stinging you. Simply avoid swatting at them, stepping on them, or otherwise coming in contact with them. Long distance insect sprays can kill stinging insects in their nests before the nests are removed.

Insects can be repelled by the use of the product Skin-So-Soft, manufactured by Avon, which may be superior to most insect repellents, The manufacturer does not advertise it or recommend it for this purpose, but guides in the Okefenokee Swamp swear by its effectiveness in repelling all sorts of stinging and biting insects. I can't recommend it over other products advertised as insect repellents, but it may be less toxic to humans.

## Insomnia

Insomnia or loss of sleep is often caused by drinking beverages containing caffeine. If you suffer from insomnia, try to avoid coffee, cola drinks and other beverages containing caffeine, or at least only take them in the morning. Caffeine is retained by the body for hours after it is taken. It has a half-life in the body of about four hours. This means that one-half of the amount of the drug that is in the body at any particular time will still be present four hours later.

Don't overlook the fact that insomnia can be caused by consumption of alcohol or prescription drugs. Consult with your doctor if you think that a prescription drug you are taking may be causing you to lose sleep. And remember that while alcohol is a sedative, excessive consumption of alcohol can produce insomnia. When alcohol's sedative effect wears off in the middle of the night, some people may awaken.

Avoid habitually using sleeping pills, because you may become addicted to them. Some people advocate taking supplements of the amino acid L-tryptophan, which has been reported to act as a natural sedative. Unfortunately, other reports indicate supplements of L-tryptophan may accelerate the aging process.

One health secret for eliminating insomnia is to get plenty of regular exercise, such as walking or working out-of-doors during the day, but not in the hours immediately preceding going to bed. This tires the muscles and helps the body to relax as the day draws to an end

Another remedy for insomnia is to avoid eating food at least two hours before bedtime and to eat light suppers instead of heavy meals.

If insomnia persists after trying the preceding health tips, try this. Upon awakening at night or experiencing insomnia, get up and stay awake throughout the remainder of the night and throughout the next day without napping. The next evening your body will be so tired that you will usually have no trouble going to sleep and staying asleep for the entire night. After this, your sleep patterns will be much more regular. If you should experience insomnia again, try the same technique. After you do this several times, your body may adjust to getting just the right amount of sleep each night without awakening.

## Itching

Itching can be caused by infections, allergic reactions, bites or drug side effects. Itching can also be caused by parasites under the skin or diseases or reactions which need medical attention.

Itching which is caused by parasites can be relieved by certain prescription drugs which should be administered after consulting a doctor. Itching from chigger or red bug bites can be relieved by applying over-the-counter medicines containing collodion or by applying heavy nail polish to the bite to block oxygen. This health secret usually relieves itching within a few minutes as the chigger dies.

Fungus infections on the skin are best treated with over-the-counter medicine containing tolnaftate.

Yeast infections in the female reproductive tract can be treated with prescription drugs, and in many cases they can be prevented with diets which are low in sugar. Yeast thrive on sugar. Another method of preventing yeast infections is to eat homemade live culture yogurt or to take freeze dried yogurt culture which is sometimes sold in capsule form.

Rectal itching may be caused by serious disease which should be treated by a physician, allergic reactions to various foods, or by prescription drugs such as antibiotics.

Itching from poison ivy is usually treated by physicians with prescription or over-the-counter medicine containing hydrocortisone, but soothing calamine lotion may also help.

### Kidney Stones

Kidney stones can be removed by surgery or, in most cases, they can be crushed without surgery by ultrasonic waves from a machine called a lithotripser. Many large medical centers have lithotripsers.

Most, but not all, kidney stones can be prevented by eating low-protein diets, drinking plenty of fluids, voiding the bladder frequently and taking adequate amounts of pyridoxine and magnesium in the diet or as supplements.

### Leg Cramps

Common muscle cramps in the legs often occur with excessive perspiration or other loss of fluid from the body which may lead to electrolyte imbalances. Consuming plenty of fluids and taking mineral supplements containing calcium and magnesium, such as the mineral dolomite, can ease common leg and foot cramps. Standing on the ball of the foot and leaning forward against a wall to stretch the cramping muscle may bring immediate relief from the cramp. Quinine preparations may relieve leg cramps.

Leg cramps which are caused by poor circulation may be a consequence of diabetes or hardening of the arteries which should be treated by a physician. Vitamin E, aspirin and niacin have all been prescribed for improving circulation in the legs, but their effectiveness is unproven and may vary from person to person.

### Lightheadedness

Lightheadedness can occur for a number of reasons that may need medical treatment or as a side effect of overexposure to vitamin D. Vitamin D overdose may happen after taking large amounts of vitamin D supplements or after sunburn. Sunburn produces excessive amounts of vitamin D as sunlight makes contact with the oil in the skin.

### Menopause

Menopause is a natural stage in a woman's life when she stops menstruating and is no longer able to give birth to children. As levels of female hormones within the body change during menopause, about 25% of all women experience very unpleasant symptoms. Menopause often causes hot flashes, irritability, personality changes, unusual amounts of perspiration, dizziness and skin sensations. During menopause, women can become more susceptible to serious diseases like diabetes, osteoporosis, heart disease and high blood pressure. Women should take special care before and during menopause to ensure continuing good health.

Vitamin E has been used successfully in controlled studies to ease the "hot flashes" and other uncomfortable side effects associated with menopause.

Calcium and vitamin D intake to guard against osteoporosis or bone thinning should be at, or 25% above, the recommended daily dietary allowance level during menopause.

Estrogen is a hormone produced naturally in women, but the amount produced decreases from the time a woman is in her late 20's or early 30's until it virtually stops at menopause. If estrogen production stops suddenly, as after a hysterectomy where the ovaries are removed, estrogen replacement therapy is especially important to moderate the hormonal imbalances in the body.

Estrogen was hailed as a wonder drug in the 1960's and given to women in large doses. Then reports linked it to cancer. Researchers now believe that estrogen replacement therapy (ERT) given in LOW doses is very effective in leveling hormonal imbalances and is safe. According to the FDA (U.S. Food and Drug Administration), estrogen treatment is safest for women who have had their wombs removed in a hysterectomy.

A National Institute of Health (NIH) study concluded that to lower the risk of heart disease women should take estrogen during mid-life, especially during menopause. The death rate from heart disease in mid-life estrogen users was 1/3 the rate in women who did not take estrogen.

All in all, taking estrogen supplements helps correct more unhealthy conditions in women who are deficient than it aggravates. Statistics show that older women who take estrogen supplements live longer and healthier lives than those who don't. Prescription drugs containing low doses of both estrogen and progesterone have fewer side effects than drugs containing estrogen alone.

A new skin patch that will allow estrogen to be given through the skin rather than with a pill may reduce some of the unwanted side effects and risks of estrogen treatment. The skin patch (called Estraderm® by Ciba-Geigy) provides doses of estrogen similar to those in a woman's body before menopause. Because the estrogen enters the body through the skin, it reduces side effects. Many women with gallbladder or liver problems cannot presently take estrogen pills, but they may benefit from the skin patch method. Estraderm® is in the final stages of research.

The FDA now says that daily estrogen supplements, taken after menopause, are an effective way of slowing down or preventing osteoporosis. Formerly, the FDA did not endorse estrogen treatment for osteoporosis. The National Institutes of Health (NIH) advisory panel says that estrogen helps the absorption and retention of calcium by the bones. When estrogen replacement therapy is started right after women stop menstruating, hip and wrist fractures can be reduced by as much as 60%, according to the NIH.

One study by Dr. Don Gambrell, Jr., at the Medical College of Georgia, concluded that estrogen given with progesterone may even protect some women against breast cancer.

Many women suffer from vaginal dryness and uncomfortable intercourse during and after menopause. Many doctors advocate estrogen replacement therapy for this. Others recommend that women who have continued sexual activity will experience fewer problems with vaginal dryness.

Limiting caffeine and alcohol intake may help reduce the undesirable symptoms of menopause. Caffeine found in products like coffee, tea, chocolate and "pepper" or "cola" soft drinks should be eliminated.

Smoking is especially harmful during or after menopause.

### Nails

Riboflavin (vitamin B2), iron, zinc, dietary protein and gelatin supplements help keep nails healthy. Zinc deficiency often shows up as white spots on the nails. Gelatin helps keep nails from becoming brittle.

### Numbness:  see Feeling, Loss of

### Osteoporosis

Osteoporosis is a condition that is found more often in women than in men. Osteoporosis causes bones to lose density and become brittle, so that they break or crush easily. Fractures of the spine, hip and wrist are common with osteoporosis. A visible sign of advanced osteoporosis is a humped back, sometimes called "dowager's hump" or "widow's hump". Humped backs caused by osteoporosis develop after loss of bone in the spine. They may cause pain, deformity and emotional hardship.

Osteoporosis usually occurs in women after menopause. There is no cure for damage already caused by osteoporosis, but good nutrition, adequate calcium and vitamin D intake, exercise and estrogen hormone replacement can prevent or slow down its development.

Calcium is needed to provide growth and strength in our bones. Our need for calcium doesn't end when we finish our last growing spurt as a teenager. Calcium is needed to maintain strong and healthy bones, to prevent hip fractures and osteoporosis. Nutritional authorities agree that most adult Americans do not consume enough calcium. The latest research suggests that moderate calcium, estrogen and, possibly, vitamin D supplementation can help prevent osteoporosis in aging women and also in aging men (minus the estrogen). Good, natural sources of calcium include: dairy products, leafy green vegetables, sunflower and sesame seeds, soybeans, corn tortillas and tofu.

Fluoride supplements in low doses may help provide stronger bones, fewer bone fractures, and less osteoporosis in older women. However, fluoride can cause side effects if too much is taken.

Large doses of the vitamin choline may cause over-absorption of phosphorus which may drive calcium out of the bones. Therefore, large doses of choline may contribute to bone degeneration and increased fractures. If large doses of choline are taken, more calcium may be needed to maintain bone strength.

Phosphorus is needed for healthy bones, but it is usually more than adequate in our diets. Taking more than the RDA of phosphorus may drive calcium out of the bones. Excessive phosphorus in the diet from soft drinks or other sources may contribute to osteoporosis and bone fractures.

Diets that are low in protein, salt and sugar may help prevent osteoporosis.

The U.S. Food and Drug Administration (FDA) says that prescribed estrogen tablets, taken daily after menopause, are an effective way of slowing down or preventing osteoporosis. A National Institute of Health (NIH) advisory panel says that estrogen helps bones to absorb and retain calcium. According to the NIH, rates of future hip and wrist fractures can be reduced by as much as 60% when estrogen replacement therapy is started soon after women stop menstruating.

## Pain

Pain is a consequence of many diseases and health problems. It can be a warning sign to seek medical help or to take steps to relieve the pain. If pain isn't diagnosed as being caused by a serious disease, it can be combated in many ways.

The obvious way to reduce pain is to avoid activities which increase the pain. A sudden sharp pain in a hand, foot, arm or a leg may be your body's way of warning you not to put pressure on that area, so that a sprain or an injury will have time to heal. Nausea and stomach pain may be a signal from your body for bedrest and fasting for a few hours, so that your body can clear up whatever is causing the upset stomach. Taking artificial steps to relieve such pain can make you think that you're better than you really are, and allow you to do things which interfere with your body's efforts to heal the cause of the pain.

Aspirin is the drug most often prescribed for relief of pain from common problems like headaches, muscle aches or muscle sprains. Aspirin not only relieves pain, but it also reduces inflammation which may accompany pain and cause pressure in the painful area. Acetaminophen, a drug which is similar to aspirin, can also relieve pain, although not quite as well as aspirin. Acetaminophen does not reduce inflammation.

L-tryptophan, an amino acid which is sold in health food stores and in vitamin and mineral sections of supermarkets or drug stores, also seems to be an effective pain reliever in recent studies. L-tryptophan seems to increase the body's production of substances in the brain which act on the brain's pleasure-pain center to lower pain signals coming from the body.

Recent studies indicate that L-tryptophan is not particularly effective against headache pain, but it may help reduce the discomfort of chronic backache and leg pain. It is hard to evaluate how much influence the "placebo" effect may have on reported pain reduction in people who take L-tryptophan.

Severe pain, such as pain from terminal cancer, is best combated by codeine, morphine or drugs similar in chemical structure to them. These drugs can be addictive or cause tolerance to develop in patients who take them, and they should not be taken for pain for a long period of time, except under extreme circumstances.

See also: **Headache,** for more information on relieving headache pain.

### Pneumonia

Pneumonia is a serious infection of the lung(s) or bronchial tubes, which can be fatal if not treated by antibiotics under a physician's care. It occurs frequently in people who have suffered from other illnesses, such as flu, and it is especially dangerous in older people.

Now there are two pneumonia vaccines which can prevent many, but not all, cases of pneumonia. Anyone at special risk for catching pneumonia, such as people who have experienced serious respiratory disease or older folks, should seriously consider taking a pneumonia vaccine. The vaccines have a low reported incidence of side effects.

### Psoriasis

Psoria.,is is a skin condition, usually found as pink or red spots with characteristic silver scaling. Psoriasis may be caused by arthritis or by hereditary or other unknown factors.

There isn't a good medical cure for psoriasis, although physicians prescribe a variety of ointments and prescription drugs in its treatment, some of which may reduce discomfort. Zinc supplements may be helpful. In a recent study, many people experienced relief and improvement in their cases of psoriasis after taking zinc supplements. The recommended daily dietary allowance for zinc is 15 mg. per day for adults.

**Ringing in the Ears:** see **Ear Noises**

## Schizophrenia

Schizophrenia is a mental illness characterized by disturbances in thinking, mood and behavior. Mild cases of schizophrenia may be characterized by loss of emotion, more severe cases by suspicion and hostility, and the most severe cases experience hallucinations or bizarre behavior.

Some physicians have found that large doses of niacin are useful in the treatment of schizophrenia. A small minority of psychiatrists use it as a treatment of first choice, but most psychiatrists think it isn't a reliable treatment. Studies by Hoffer and Osmond, with the Provincial Mental Hospital patients of Saskatchewan in the 1950's, indicated that their niacin treatment was effective. But other later control studies indicate that it was less effective than treatment with phenothiazine drugs for severe cases.

In some cases of schizophrenia, niacin appears to be better than treatment with powerful tranquilizers, and it has fewer severe side effects. Many schizoid personalities or moderately severe, long-term chronic, paranoid schizophrenics, for which it works best, have improved dramatically after taking 1,500 to 3,000 mg. of niacin in 3 daily doses of 500 to 1,000 mg. per dose. Niacin may help schizophrenics by increasing the body's production of serotonin, a neurohormone (nervous system hormone) or by helping to rid the body of by-products of faulty neurohormone metabolism.

In severe cases of schizophrenia, niacin may not be enough to combat the illness; then, potent phenothiazine tranquilizers like Thorazine® are used to block the body's production of dopamine, another neurohormone. Unfortunately, Thorazine® can have serious side effects. Approximately 10% of people who take large doses of Thorazine® suffer from uncontrollable, irreversible muscle spasms called tardive dyskinesia.

Large doses of niacin should only be taken under the advice of a physician. They should never be taken on an empty stomach, because they could cause serious side effects such as upset stomach or even ulcers. One alarming but relatively harmless side effect of taking niacin is a reddening or flushing of the skin for an hour or so after taking large doses of the vitamin. The flushing reaction usually disappears after the body becomes accustomed to the continued large doses of niacin.

## Senility

Senility is memory loss, disorientation, confusion and loss of reasoning ability with advancing age. There is a difference between the natural slowing of our reaction time with advancing age and being senile. Only about 5% of older Americans suffer from true senility.

Alzheimer's disease causes people to lose their memory and become senile. High levels of aluminum have been found in the brains of people who have Alzheimer's disease. Aluminum can get into the body from drinking water, baking powder, flour and cake mixes, pancake mixes, table salt, salad dressings, frozen dough, self-rising flour, processed cheese, some pickled cucumbers, nondairy creamers, buffered aspirin, antacids, anti-diarrhea products, douches, aluminum pots and pans, deodorants, skin creams, lipsticks, lotions, and hemorrhoid creams.

Some researchers theorize that drinking three glasses of skim milk per day or taking fluoride supplements may interfere with the uptake of aluminum into the body and help prevent Alzheimer's disease from developing.

However, avoiding aluminum may not help prevent Alzheimer's disease. Some researchers think that aluminum accumulation in the brain is a byproduct of the disease and not its cause. Good nutrition and other practices that promote good health may help prevent senility. A British doctor, Roy Hullin, found lower levels of zinc in people who were senile than in people who were not senile. Dr. Hullin feels that the elderly do not get enough zinc in their diets. Zinc is plentiful in meats and seafood.

Pantothenic acid (Vitamin B5) supplements may improve symptoms of senility and depression when taken with other B vitamins.

## Sex Drive

Reduced sex drive is often associated with hormonal changes which occur as a consequence of aging. Lack of estrogen after menopause may cause dryness in the vagina which makes intercourse uncomfortable. Estrogen supplements may help restore normal sexual activity in post menopausal women.

Certain vitamins, taken to excess, may interfere with the sex drive. Vitamin D overdose may cause decreased sex drive. Reduced sexual function may be caused by overdoses of vitamin E.

See also: **Impotence.**

## Skin Problems

People's ages are often judged by the condition of their skins. If it is smooth and elastic, the person is assumed to be young. But if it is wrinkled and leathery, the person is assumed to be old. Our face and hands are affected most by factors which age the skin, and people notice them first.

The chief causes of excessive skin wrinkling are smoking, exposure to sunlight, and reduced hormone levels, especially in women after menopause when estrogen levels drop drastically.

Most smokers have skin that looks twenty years older than their natural age would indicate. Giving up smoking can restore much of the vitality and elasticity to skin in ex-smokers.

Excessive exposure to the sun from sun bathing, working or playing sports in the sun without protection causes the skin to become tanned and leathery. Wearing hats and other protective clothing and covering unprotected areas with sunscreens or sun-blockers can protect the skin.

Women who have had hysterectomies, or who are at or beyond menopause, may discover that their prescribed hormone supplements keep their skin looking youthful.

*Dry, itchy skin* plagues many older people. With aging, the skin often becomes dry, as the oil glands produce less. Cleansing with soap in a long, hot bath actually makes the problem <u>worse</u>. Bathe, shower and wash in cool water to keep your skin moist. Use a soap containing glycerin to keep your skin from drying out. Bath oils make your skin feel good, but they make the tub very slippery and are dangerous to use. Rubbing your face with a facecloth or using a facial mask will help remove dead skin and stimulate the growth of new skin

Early symptoms of niacin (Vitamin B3) deficiency include skin sores or a skin rash resembling a heat rash with painful red spots. The skin may have a red appearance like a sunburn. In a severe niacin deficiency, the skin may become dry, scaly and inflexible.

Itching can be a sign of vitamin D overdose, like that which happens after a sunburn.

*Dry, cracked or blemished skin* can be a sign of vitamin C or vitamin A deficiency. Vitamin A maintains the smoothness, health and functioning of the skin and the mucous membranes. Vitamin A also helps build body protein and promotes the growth of body tissues. Derivatives of vitamin A are used as acne treatments.

An extreme overdose of Vitamin A can cause dry skin or peeling of the skin.

*Photosensitivity* is an exaggerated redness of the skin after brief sun exposure. Redness, swelling, hives, and itching are symptoms of photosensitivity. If your skin is photosensitive, it usually reacts to the sun more quickly and severely than normal. Some drugs actually can cause photosensitivity. These medications include: tetracyclines, thiazide diuretics, antidiabetics, oral contraceptives, antipsychotics, antidepressants, antihistamines, anticancer drugs, corticosteroids and psoralens. Non-drug products that can also cause photosensitivity include: coal tar products, coal tar dyes, musk fragrance, some perfumes, some cosmetics and even some sunscreens.

*Poor skin color and appearance* may be caused by zinc deficiency. Zinc helps the growth and repair of the body and helps the B vitamins work properly.

*Wrinkled and sagging skin* has been reported as a side effect of fluoride taken at, or above, the recommended level.

Vitamin E supplementation may reduce skin wrinkles.

**Sleeplessness:** see **Insomnia**

**Smell, Loss of**

Loss of smell can be a symptom of sinus infection or other serious disease that needs medical attention. It may also be a symptom of vitamin A deficiency or zinc deficiency. Liver, eggs and whole milk products are good food sources of vitamin A. Carotene, which is converted by the body into vitamin A, is found in fruits and vegetables, especially yellow vegetables such as carrots. Many vitamins are destroyed in cooking food, but carotene is released when vegetables are cooked. Thus, cooked vegetables are better sources of carotene than raw vegetables.

Liver, seafood, dairy products, meat and eggs are good sources of zinc. Vegetable products are poor sources of zinc. Whole wheat and other whole grain products contain zinc in a less available form than animal products. There is very little zinc in most water supplies.

## Smoking

Health consequences of smoking include loss of teeth from depletion of vitamin C in the gums, excessive wrinkling which makes smokers look years older than they really are, loss of physical stamina, loss of appetite, greatly increased rates of lung disease, heart disease and high blood pressure. Smoking causes emphysema, which is a loss of the elasticity in the lungs, and chronic bronchitis, in many cases. Throat and larynx problems also often occur.

Smoking has social consequences. It creates stale odors which get into furniture and hair. Smoking leaves stains on teeth and causes bad breath. It makes many non-smokers uncomfortable.

Smokers continue smoking even when they realize it is bad for their health, because nicotine is one of the most addictive substances known to man. It is extremely difficult for a smoker to quit smoking because of the physical craving for nicotine which is found in tobacco products.

Using other tobacco products may be less harmful, overall, than smoking cigarettes, but smoking cigars, pipes and chewing smokeless tobacco greatly increases risks for cancer of the throat, mouth, tongue and neck.

Most people can't give up smoking without determination and help from everyone who cares for the smoker. Withdrawal from nicotine can be eased by a prescription drug called Nicorette® which slowly releases a measured dose of nicotine into the system to reduce physical craving for tobacco products. Withdrawal from nicotine may also be eased by taking half a teaspoon of bicarbonate of soda in a glass of water two or three times a day. Apparently, the bicarbonate of soda helps hold nicotine in the system and reduce withdrawal symptoms by giving the body more time to adapt to withdrawal.

Once a smoker has successfully withdrawn from tobacco for two weeks, most withdrawal symptoms should pass.

Regular aerobic exercise such as running, walking, playing tennis, swimming, bike riding, hard physical labor and association with non-smokers help in giving up smoking and resisting temptation to return to smoking.

**Strep Throat:** see **Throat, Strep**

**Stroke Prevention**

A stroke occurs when a blood vessel in the brain ruptures or becomes blocked by a clot. Strokes are closely related to coronary heart disease and atherosclerosis, so things that help prevent them may also help prevent strokes.

Strokes are found more often in areas of the country where the water is soft, containing few minerals other than sodium. The "stroke belt", close to the Atlantic coast in Georgia and South Carolina, is an area where the water is soft.

People who live in areas of the country where the water is hard, containing minerals such as calcium, magnesium, and selenium, have lower rates of strokes. Adding these minerals to the diet in the form of mineral supplements or drinking mineral water may help to prevent strokes in areas where the water is soft.

See also: **Coronary Heart Disease.**

## Swelling In Feet and Legs

Swelling in feet and legs may be a symptom of kidney disease or heart disease so see your doctor. Swelling in the feet and legs in women may be caused by hormonal imbalances, especially at the end of the monthly cycle. Supplements of the B vitamin, pyridoxine, and magnesium may help prevent premenstrual tension and bloating.

See also: **Coronary Heart Disease** and **Blood Pressure, High**

147

## Tardive Dyskinesia

Tardive dyskinesia is an irreversible deterioration of the central nervous system which causes uncontrollable muscle spasms in approximately 10% of the people who take phenothiazine tranquilizers for a long period of time.

Niacin, other B vitamins such as choline, and vitamin C may be useful in preventing the development of tardive dyskinesia in mental patients who are taking a powerful phenothiazine tranquilizer such as Thorazine®.

There have been no controlled scientific studies in this area, but some physicians who prescribe large doses of vitamins in addition to phenothiazine tranquilizers in their psychiatric practices have reported seeing no cases of tardive dyskinesia among their long-term patients.

## Taste, Loss of

Loss of taste is often closely related to loss of smell. The taste buds can distinguish sweetness, saltiness and bitterness, but finer distinctions of taste are related to the sense of smell. Smoking or use of other tobacco products can cause problems with taste by damaging the tastebuds.

See also:  **Smell, Loss of.**

## Teeth

Small doses of fluoride help prevent cavities and harden tooth enamel, but overdoses of fluoride at, or above, the recommended daily dietary allowance can cause chalky, white areas on the teeth.  Severe overdoses of fluoride can cause brown stains and pitting of teeth. Phosphorus, calcium, vitamin A and vitamin D are essential or important for the development of strong teeth.  Vitamin C is necessary for the maintenance of healthy gums, which help prevent gum infections and loss of teeth.

See also:  **Dental Problems.**

## Teeth Grinding (Bruxism)

Taking pantothenic acid (vitamin B5) is claimed to lower the incidence of bruxism, the grinding of teeth, during sleep.

## Throat Problems

Sore throat can be a symptom of a serious illness or a serious illness in itself and should be treated by a physician, especially if it is accompanied by a skin rash, fever, headache, vomiting, stomach pain, or swollen glands. Any sore throat in a person with a history of rheumatic fever or kidney disease should be treated by a physician.

If your physician agrees, sore throats can be treated naturally by using a salt water gargle. Salt water gargles may work as well as antibiotics because many sore throats are caused by bacterial infections. Simply dissolve a teaspoon of salt in a cup of warm water and gargle for 10 or 15 seconds, three or four times a day.

To help recovery, also drink plenty of fluids and get plenty of rest.

**Throat, Strep**

Strep throat is a particular type of throat infection caused by streptococci. A positive diagnosis of strep throat can be made by a physician by taking a swab from the back of the throat and culturing the mucus from the swab.

Strep throats may cause serious complications, including rheumatic fever, which may lead to rheumatic heart disease.

Persistent strep throat infections may be caused by spreading germs back and forth between family members or pets. Once a person has been successfully treated for strep throat, it is a good idea to discard all toothbrushes and to periodically disinfect new toothbrushes with a dilute hydrogen peroxide solution and then rinse the toothbrushes off before using.

Recently, researchers have discovered that pets can be carriers of strep throat and reinfect family members, especially small children who may come into close contact with pets.

Recurrent strep throat infections should be treated by:

1.  Checking all family members to make sure that they are not carriers.

2.  Discarding all old toothbrushes and periodically disinfecting new toothbrushes.

3.  Frequently changing sheets, pillowcases, hand towels and washcloths, and allowing only one family member to use one towel or washcloth at a time.

4.  If all else fails, checking the family pet.

**Tinnitus:** see **Ear Noises**

**Toothache:** see **Dental Problems**

**Toxemia of Pregnancy**

Toxemia of pregnancy, also called eclampsia, and in its early stages called pre-eclampsia, is a life-threatening condition which occurs late in pregnancy. True eclampsia or pre-eclampsia should be treated by a physician, but recent studies indicate that the condition may be prevented by proper nutrition during pregnancy.

Studies of pregnant women who have lots of magnesium, calcium and high quality protein in their diets, indicate that these nutrients, and perhaps other nutrients, can help prevent cases of toxemia of pregnancy. Milk or milk products, whole grain products and vegetables are excellent natural sources of these nutrients. Mineral supplements may be helpful.

### Ulcers

Stomach ulcers can occur for a variety of reasons. Ulcers are uncommon in people who eat a diet that contains a lot of dietary fiber, such as fiber found in whole grain products. Although whole grain products can't cure stomach ulcers, in many cases they can help prevent their recurrence once healed, according to a recent scientific study.

Stomach ulcers can be treated quite successfully by two prescription drugs, Tagamet® and Zantac®. Zantac® has fewer side effects than Tagamet®, but it is more expensive. Both drugs shut off the flow of stomach acid which prevents stomach ulcers from healing. Healing usually takes place within a few weeks of taking one of these drugs.

Another treatment for ulcers that some doctors prescribe is to take an antacid every hour while awake as well as upon rising once during the middle of the night. This treatment can be effective, but it is hard for patients to be completely faithful in doing something every hour on the hour.

People with ulcers should avoid foods which cause stomach pain. Meat, hot foods and drinks, spicy foods, acidic foods, and hard fibrous foods, such as raw carrots or popcorn, may aggravate ulcers. Soft foods are well tolerated, and foods containing fiber are well tolerated if the fiber is finely ground whole wheat flour, oat flour or oatmeal.

### Varicose Veins

Varicose veins are greatly enlarged blood vessels, usually in the legs. Blood flow slows as it passes through varicose veins, and clots may form. Varicose veins are usually treated by doctors by prescribing support hose or by surgical removal. Support hose, in most cases, may work as well as surgery and present fewer risks.

The chief cause of varicose veins is a low-fiber diet which causes a hard stool. Resultant constipation exerts considerable pressure against the veins from the legs which pass through the abdominal cavity. The longer the transit time, (time taken for food to be digested and excreted as feces) the more prolonged the pressure. This pressure makes valves in the veins, which prevent blood from flowing backward, open up and the veins balloon out.

Dr. Dennis Burkitt of the British Medical Research Council reported in the medical journal Lancet on a large study of 1,000 subjects of varying ethnic groups, including British boarding school children, rural African villagers, and British vegetarians. His results showed that the greater the removal of fiber from the diet, the smaller the stool and the longer the transit time of food through the intestine.

The following are various studies relating to varicose veins from areas where people eat diets high in dietary fiber like bran, which is found in whole grain products.

1. Over a three-year period 11,462 patients were admitted to a hospital in the Zululand Reserve in South Africa. In addition, the hospital treated 103,857 outpatients. Of all these, there were only three reported cases of

varicose veins. (In a similar U.S. study, we'd expect to see well over 10,000 cases).

2. A worker in another African hospital studied 30,000 out-patients and found only one case of varicosities.

3. Dr. Burkitt personally examined 4,000 adults in Central Africa and detected only five cases of varicose veins.

4. A questionnaire sent to doctors in 114 hospitals in Africa showed that 87% of the doctors estimated that they saw less than five patients per year with varicose veins.

5. Questionnaires sent to hospitals in India and Pakistan in areas where high-fiber diets are eaten indicated a similar low incidence of varicose veins.

It seems evident from such studies that a diet high in fiber may offer protection against varicose veins, whereas a diet low in fiber can be linked with a high percentage of varicose veins in a population.

### Yeast Infections

"Yeast infections" means infections by yeast-like fungi such as candida albicans. Yeast infections may occur after antibiotic treatment for bacterial infection. Thrush, an infection of the mouth especially found in infants that is characterized by white patches, ulcers, fever and gastrointestinal upset, is caused by candida albicans. Vaginal infections and skin infections such as "jock itch" can be caused by candida albicans or similar fungi. Persistent inner ear infections in children may be caused by fungi.

Many other conditions such as anxiety, crying, depression, bloating, diarrhea, constipation, indigestion, acne, hives, headaches, nasal, sinus and bronchial allergies, menstrual disorders, decreased sex drive, or premenstrual tension may be caused by yeast infections.

Treatment for yeast infections is simple and quite effective. There are prescription drugs to combat yeast infections, including Nystatin® which prevents the growth of yeast in the digestive tract and helps prevent the spread of yeast infections from the digestive tract to other areas of the body. Nystatin® has almost no side effects, since it is not absorbed into the body. Any side effects associated with Nystatin® are usually caused by the presence of dead yeast in the digestive tract for a few days until they are expelled.

Yeast infections can be combated naturally by avoiding sugars, such as sugary drinks, candy, or many processed foods containing sugar and also by avoiding eating excessive carbohydrates like white flour products. Taking supplements of acidophilus lactobacillus cultures or active yogurt  which is cultured at home can help by displacing harmful yeast with benign organisms.

## In Closing

The hidden health secrets in this book are based on reports of "natural" methods of healing, but don't overlook the supernatural power of God from whence all healing comes. If you put your faith and trust in Him by following His son, Jesus Christ, He will answer your prayers for healing according to His will. If you would like to know more about how to have eternal life through Jesus Christ, please write to:   FC&A, Dept. JC 86, 103 Clover Green, Peachtree City, Georgia 30269.

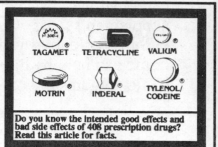

# "Natural Healing Encyclopedia"

## An Encyclopedia of Natural Cures and HealthTips

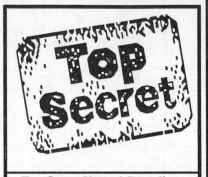

**Top Secret Natural Remedies for What Ails You**

**(Atlanta, GA)**
FC&A, a nearby Peachtree City, Georgia health publisher announced today the release of a new, $9.95 book for the general public, *"Natural Healing Encyclopedia"*.

**Look at Some of the Secrets Revealed in This New Book.**

- Alzheimer's Disease from your cookware? Check your pots and pans.
- Chest pain is directly related to heart disease severity. Right? Not always.
- Sleeplessness. Causes and common-sense remedies.
- Feeling tired? This simple remedy helps many.
- Looking older? "Aging symptoms" may only be a side effect of a prescription drug you're taking.
- Inner ear noises could be from a lack of these vitamins in your diet.
- A nutritional supplement to help poor memory.
- Find out what the back of your hand has to do with a toothache.
- Wrinkles are unavoidable, right? Wrong! The way we sleep and talk can make the difference.
- Counting sheep to help you sleep isn't just an old tale.
- A Q-tip® may actually help you get rid of the hiccups.
- Relieve leg cramps with this simple trick.
- When you eat can help you lose weight.
- Fluoride can help prevent tooth decay — we know that. But did you know that it may also help fight a common disease of aging?
- Taking laxatives? Try this simple, natural remedy.
- Ways to avoid life-threatening blood clots.
- High blood pressure? Natural, drug-free ways to bring it down.
- Oatmeal isn't only for breakfast. Find out how to use it to help relieve itching from poison ivy.
- Rubber gloves will protect your hands, right? No. They can actually do harm.
- Find out what freckles and oatmeal have in common.
- Vitamins and minerals that may actually slow down aging.
- See how a tennis ball can stop your mate from snoring.
- Secrets to revitalize your hair, nails and skin.
- See how some people treat asthma symptoms with coffee and cheese.
- How to guard yourself against widow's hump or osteoporosis.
- This common herb can keep your breath fresh naturally.
- Soaking in this breakfast drink can help get rid of body odor.
- Your mother's chicken soup — why it really helps colds.
- Strokes are totally unrelated to heart disease. Right? Wrong.
- Got a bad cough? You might try this common beverage.
- How garlic may help fight against diabetes.
- Is something you're eating or taking causing your indigestion? How to find out.
- How to get rid of corns and calluses — for good.
- A common headache medicine that often causes dizziness.
- Age spots? Apply this fruit juice, and they disappear.
- Fast relief for a toothache.

**Free With Order.**
**Don't Wait, Order Now.**
You must cut out and return this notice with your order. Copies will not be accepted!
Order *"Natural Healing Encyclopedia"* now! Tear out and return this notice with your name and address and a check for $9.95 + $2.00 shipping and handling to our following address: FC&A, Dept. SAZ-7, 103 Clover Green, Peachtree City, GA 30269.
Save! Return this notice with $19.90 + $2.00 for two books. (No extra shipping and handling charges).
You get a free gift and a no-time-limit guarantee of satisfaction or your money back. ©FC&A 1987